BUDDHISM FOR BEGINNERS

CLEAR AND SIMPLE GUIDE TO INTRODUCE YOU TO THE BUDDHISM AND ZEN TEACHINGS, DISCOVER THE YOGA MEDITATION, THE SUTRAS PHILOSOPHY AND THE SECRET OF DEEP RELAXATION WITH YOGA NIDRA

AURORA COOPER

ISBN: 9798647076298

Contents

Introduction

On December 2007, I embarked on a mission to escape the boring winter and have a break from the shadows of my past. I chose to travel to Thailand... just to appreciate and learn more about the kind of rice that I always loved to cook that came from Southeast Asia. Exactly the kind of spontaneous and crazy backpacking trips I love.

One sunny day while I was walking down towards one of the rice fields, I saw a group of five people gathered down by a tree in what was plainly clear to me as monks with the simplest form of being – no hair, no shoes, loose robes, no chair or stool. They manifested a gentle mien and serene appearance and seemed unperturbed by the chaotic world around them.

They were very simple, taking on a clean diet of boiled rice and some vegetables, using Thai sticks, which appeared as just a pair of thicker and more elongated toothpicks. No spoons, and still no plates as they were being served food on some kind of roundish basket on which a fitting piece of green banana leaf was spread under the food.

It was such a simplicity and calm that baffled me. It created in me an inner desire to understand how they lived their lives in a way that manifested such a compelling authenticity of peace, harmony and serenity. I started seeking knowledge about their ways of life and started practicing the little things that I learned from them. Well, it did take me some time before I discovered that I was already in the middle of practicing Buddhism.

Buddhism basics

Buddhism refers to the practice of teachings of Buddha. However, for purposes of a fast grasp of Buddhism, let's look at what Buddhism is and what Buddhism is not, in order to set ourselves on the right knowledge pedestal.

What Buddhism is not:

Is not a religion – Buddhism shares with major religions one common thing: doctrine. However, unlike others, it's not a religion per se. Though still, there are those who have opted to refer to it or practice it as religion. What used to make me fear practicing Buddhism was my wrongly held belief that Buddhism was a weird and bizarre religion that was incompatible with Western ways of living. While in Thailand, under the tutelage of a Buddhist monk, I came to learn how Buddha encouraged his followers not to blindly follow, but arrive at their own truths about his teachings. This made me gain courage to explore more of his wisdom. No religion grants you this freedom to arrive at your own truths about it except Buddhism, which is simply 'a religion that is non-religious'. My increased awareness of Buddhism granted me the first step to pursuing my liberty by not rigidly holding onto any religion in particular, but exploring all religions as much as I could in search of truth without being ensnared by traps of dogmatism. Indeed, I was truly liberated.

Chapter 1.
Core Concept

Paying on this book the whole Buddhist teaching would be impossible. However, it is doable to get familiar inside the basic concept that you'll be able to apply in your health.

Then again, this is not an unexpected transformation. You might even get contrasting some of these concepts, mainly if are derived from a belief that disagrees with all the claims with the Buddhist practice.

A. Life and also the Material World

The notion of Buddhism in life and the material world revolves around the belief in reincarnation. Here, the repetitive cycle of birth, death after which rebirth is named the Samsara. This cycle often happens inside the six plains of existence. Renewal on a certain plain is usually derived from the Karma, or the deeds sowed as seeds by a person within a lifetime. These seeds may do tremendous or bad. Consequences of these seeds could happen within precisely the same life if the seed is sown or upon the following cycle of rebirth. Karma is influenced only through the individual who planted his or her seed. This idea of Karma often results in ignorance from what could be the true enlightenment if anyone is not able to continue with the path to nirvana.

Rebirth then becomes the entire process of successive lifetimes. These lifetimes all start in the moment of conception towards the moment of death. A sentient being can be reborn in any of the six plains (or five plains depending in the branch being followed). These plains are the Naraka, Preta, Animal Plain, Human Plain, Asura, and Deva. Each succession is relying on cause and effect regarding the sowing of the seeds of Karma.

Naraka is the realm comparable to what other beliefs define as hell. It has to be understood though that there can be various forms of Naraka depending on the being that's reborn in this plain.

Preta, on the other hand, maybe the ghost realm. It sometimes shares its existence with the human field thus making the beings within these realms capable of interacting collectively in certain circumstances.

The animal realm shares the same reality in the human field. Still, the beings within these realms are viewed different life forms. This concept could technically be the way to obtain the idea of most Buddhist vegetarians not to eat meat.

The human realm is technically the realm where you are reading this article book as in the moment. Alternatively, in a very sensitive, it could be the realm the location where the author wrote the written text you are reading basing on Buddhist beliefs.

The Asura realm could be the plain for lesser deities for the people beings in a position to reach a specific a higher level of enlightenment. Still, this plain could be home to demons also which may technically be argued capably to reach an enlightened state in their own right.

The Deva realm could be the plain committed to the deities, angels, and spirits who can attain the highest type of enlightenment.

B. The Suffering (Causes and Solutions)

It is time and energy to see the causes with the suffering inside the human realm basing on Buddhist beliefs. To indeed see why part, you need to learn two central teachings.

First, you must learn about The Four Noble Truths. According to Buddhism, suffering (Dukkha) might be explained through its causes and also the ways that it can be eased and then improved. The first truth then focuses on the reality that suffering exists. A person must realize that there is undoubtedly suffering in your life as a way to truly understand it.

The second truth is the undeniable fact that suffering has their origins. Once pain is accepted, it's time for it to seek out its source. Once the background is available, it will be clearer why it causes the sufferings of life.

The third truth deals while using the proven fact that each supply of suffering carries a solution. You must accept first that any problems can be ended and therefore it is just not eternal. In a feeling, it works with keeping hope being a fact and necessity in your life.

The last truth reveals the route to locating the solution for that suffering.

The second Buddhist with instructions on a need to learn will be the Noble Eight Fold Path. This teaching can help you accept The Four Noble Truths of life. The eightfold is divided into three divisions, each having specific folds under his or her instructions.

The first division relates to wisdom. The first fold under this division could be the Right View. It means you need to view reality as it can be and never the way appears to get based on how you want to notice. The next fold will be the Right Intention it indicates you need to know what you need with regards to rejecting and thus freedom from a preference of reality.

The next division concentrates on ethical conduct. The first fold here could be the Right Speech. This fold indicates that everything has to be spoken should be true yet mustn't hurt, euphemisms should come in handy. The next fold is the Right Action which states that you must act in the best way you cannot hurt anyone. The last fold in this division will be the Right Livelihood. It should speak for itself but to clarify it is finding your ends meet in techniques cannot hurt or compromise other beings or Lives.

The last division may be the concentration. The leading fold with this division is the Right Effort, meaning you must have the will to improve yourself further and not dwell about the level in which you are not going to continue. Next fold is the Right Mindfulness. This fold of Right Mindfulness states a person with the current scenario in your life without trying to hide from yourself any information on whether it can be good or bad. The last fold could be the Right Concentration that states that you should hold power to concentrate your efforts by combining the applications of all the folds into one existence in your health. Right meditation may be a way of amplifying it further.

C. Reasons and nature of Existence

This goal is also the fact drives everyone to get with an answer to the question of what makes someone happy. In reality though, if your answer is using the Buddhist tradition, happiness can only be defined through the individual that asked the question. One the definition becomes concrete then a road to contentment is see-through. The nature of existing then can be determined now since anyone who asked already knows what he wants to do in life.

The next step for you then is usually to become see your face who will likely be thinking.

D. Liberation

Now that you be aware of question you'll want to think about it is possible to start to try to liberate yourself through the bonds which are hindering you. You are given a blueprint to begin things out.

Chapter 2.
What is Buddhism

Hello! You must be the kind of person who is eager to learn new things every day. After all, why else would you choose this book?

You must be curious about Buddhism. You might have heard of it from somewhere, such as on social media or from a friend who is passionate about its teachings.

You might also have heard about the many ways it has helped those who find their true purpose in life, or – at the very least – find peace and calm in the midst of a seemingly fast-paced and stressful world.

A million questions might be swimming in your brain concerning Buddhism. In a while, they will be answered.

First, do take comfort in being here right now: reading this book and acquiring the knowledge that can help you find true happiness in everyday life.

Look around you and notice how your body has naturally kept you alive. Your lungs continue to breathe without you having to tell them to do so. Your eyelids blink automatically to keep your eyes moist and protected.

Your blood continues to flow underneath your skin, oblivious to your surroundings and thoughts.

Also, notice how you are able to comprehend the words on this page. Is that not something to be grateful for? Take a moment to consider this thought.

Are you still here? Hopefully yes, because now let us answer what may be the first question in your mind: What is Buddhism?

What is Buddhism?

Would it surprise you to know that Buddhism is not a religion? At least, not in the sense wherein it is an institution that dictates how one should believe in a divine power. Many people make that mistake and avoid Buddhism because they believe it to be contrary to the teachings of their church. However, you can practice Buddhism in conjunction with your personal belief and religion, or as a complement to it.

In fact, there is no deity to be worshipped, although you might wonder why some seem to be worshipping the statues of the Buddha. While there indeed are those who worship his image (and erroneously so), true Buddhists merely pay respect to the memory of the Buddha. They neither worship nor pray to him. The Buddha himself is a guide and teacher for those that seek the path to enlightenment. The altars that you see in a Buddhist temple are inspirational and remind Buddhists of the path that they have chosen to walk. The colors of the decoration of a Buddhist temple are indeed made up of colors that are easily seen by the eye and the Buddha statue is there as a guide to your meditative process.

Many people who wake up each morning with the intention of practicing Buddhist teachings find inspiration from the gentle image of the Buddha. It is not unlike finding your motivation from the words of a successful person. His peaceful and meditative image can help you understand and remember the teachings you are following when life becomes stressful, and your mind begins to run off course. Thus, it follows that creating a meditative area and adorning it with a Buddha statue or other inspirational items is common for westerners.

Buddhism is a way of life that leads to the discernment of true reality. Its teachings center on developing your ability to be mindful of your thoughts, actions, and surroundings. All these lead to a life that is in tune with nature and your true self. You may find it hard to understand at first, but everything that happens in your life is dictated by your thoughts and when you meditate, you get a clearer look at what needs to change in your world, as well as learning more about who you are in relation to the world that you live in or even the body that you inhabit.

The practices of Buddhism – including meditation and yoga – are meant to help you unlearn your preconceived notions of yourself and the world. They serve as your guide towards embracing such qualities as kindness, love, true wisdom, and awareness. Over the course of our youth, we are taught society values and these may not run in line with true values which is why this reminder is needed. Look at the uncertainty in the world, and at the bottom of it, you will always find a line of thought that leads you to the unhappiness that you experience. This may be biased toward certain members of society or it may indeed be a lack of self-worth brought on by your interaction with society.

Those who continually walk the path of Buddhism usually find themselves achieving the state of "perfect enlightenment." In other words, they become a "Buddha." A Buddha is a being who has been able to see the nature of life as it truly is. The enlightened being then continues to live life fully, all the while upholding the principles that are in line with this vision. Since this philosophy may question your current motivation, your beliefs and your way of life, you need to be open-minded enough to learn because the teachings are very thorough. To reach enlightenment, you need to be able to let go of values that may at the current time be fundamental to who you are.

The idea of enlightenment can be broken down into two simple forms, the mind, and the self. The mind is that constant voice that has been molded and constructed based on the world around you in this life. Self is that inner being that is separate from the meat of your body and does not change based on any teachings or experiences that life brings you. Your real self is what can be understood to travel from life to life during reincarnation. In different belief systems, these are given names, such as the soul, though what name you give it isn't important. It is merely important that you recognize that these two parts of you exist and that, if you are unhappy in your life, the harmony or balance is missing and that's where Buddhism helps you to align these values so that both parts of you are in harmony with each other.

Each and every living being has the opportunity to become enlightened in each life they live. There is no set course or prewritten script for your life. Karma plays a part in deciding the circumstances in which you will be born into from life to life, but your own spiritual and mental ambition are what drives each person to take one step closer to full enlightenment.

However, things get interesting here, because when you follow the path of Buddhism, you do not have an "end goal." It is a paradox for one to declare that they are going to practice Buddhism in order to reach enlightenment.

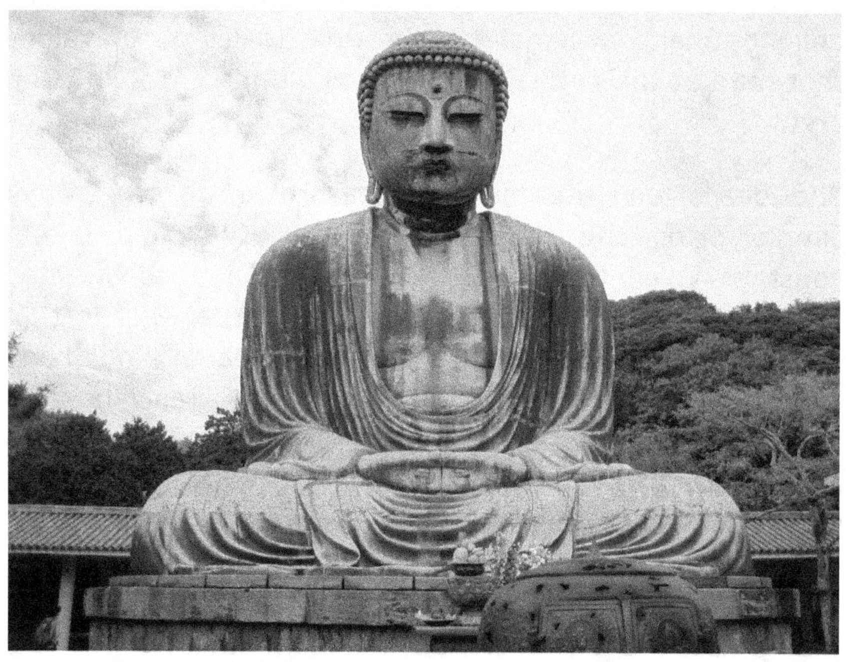

Who is The Buddha?

The word "Buddha" translates to "the enlightened one" or "the awakened being." It refers to any being who has achieved this state. However, you might be curious to know about the first Buddha.

According to legend, the first Buddha was named Siddhartha Gautama. Many believe that he was born around 563 B.C. in a land that is now found in Nepal. It is said that The Buddha was born a royal, shielded from the suffering of the kingdom of his father, who built a grand palace around him void of religion or human suffering. The King created an entire world inside those castle walls and, as his son grew, led him to believe that the world was one of happiness, empathy, and joy. The King was told by seers when the prince was born that he would either be a great warrior or a spiritual leader.

Later in his life, after he had married and was raised, he ventured out into the world and saw the truth of humanity. He met an old man and found that all people age, and eventually die.

At the age of twenty-nine, he found that neither his power nor his fortune brought him true happiness, and he wanted to understand the world outside of the palace walls.

Therefore, what he did was he set out to explore as many religions across the world as he could to find the answer to the question that we all ask ourselves, "Where can one find happiness?" He tried many ways including fasting and when he found that fasting was not helping him in the way that he thought it might, he decided to meditate on the problems that he faced. While others still practiced going without food and had thought that Siddhartha had given up the practice, he had in fact taken himself on another route – one that would lead him to enlightenment.

Several years into his spiritual pilgrimage, the Buddha discovered "The Middle Path" while meditating under the

Bodhi tree. This path is a way of balance, not of extremism, which he found only through trial and error. He sat for days under that Bodhi tree seeking the answers he had initially set out to find. During this meditation, Siddhartha had to face the evil demon known as Mara, who threatened to stand in the way of his Buddha status. He looked to the earth for guidance and the land answered by banishing Mara and allowing Siddhartha to reach full enlightenment. Such discernment led him to achieve the perfect state of enlightenment. After this life-changing experience, the Buddha then lived the rest of his days sharing what he had discovered. The followers of the Buddha's teachings called his principles the Dharma, or "Truth."

It is thought that Buddha or anyone who reaches the state of perfect enlightenment in their lifetime no longer continues on the circle of rebirth. Instead, the Buddha is thought to sit outside of constant reincarnation and sends teachings and guidance to those searching for their own freedom of self. They no longer have to sit through what Buddhists believe to be an endless cycle of suffering known as life.

When you hear the word suffering, you may have images of pain and anger come into your mind, but in Buddhism, they believe that all life is suffering. As humans, we feel the pain of loss, the emotions of sadness, happiness, disappointment, and so on. These emotions are manifestations of our mind, and they do not come from our inner selves. Because they do not come from our true selves, they are thought of as suffering. These are false feelings created by the meat of our brains, programmed into us by what our societal view has taught us. The way forward was through following the Noble Eightfold Path and this allowed people to be closer to the potential of enlightenment.

Currently, Buddhism is increasingly becoming a popular way of life for millions of people, across the world. Even those in the Western countries seek to follow The Middle Path because they find that it speaks to their heart. There is also the fact that traditional medicines do very little for the status quo. For example, if you are depressed or if you are unable to deal with the feelings that you have, scientists have established that the Buddhist way offers you a better and more permanent solution to your problems. Medical findings that explored the relationship between the Buddhist way and the way that the brain operated found that Buddhist monks were able to simultaneously use the creative side of the brain and the calculating side of the brain and that they were, therefore more open to creativity.

In a world where everything is always in motion, constantly forcing us to move forward at a quicker and more rapid pace, many people feel the loss of their connection with nature. Though nature is all around us, even in the major cities, what we have done to change the pure form of Earth, creates a disconnect from our minds. In Buddhism, you are connected to every natural thing in this world, and by practicing the teachings of it, you are brought back to that connection. This is an enormous draw for millions of people all over the world. You can think of it as connecting back to your roots.

If you are unsure of what this means, you only have to look to see what happens when you go somewhere that you find to be inspiring. The feelings that you experience don't just come from the external stimuli. They come from your inner self-recognizing the joy that lies in that ever moving thing called nature. We celebrate the changing of the seasons and the weather and get up close and personal with nature in an attempt to find ourselves.

Another reason why Buddhism is widespread is the fact that the Buddha never claimed to be a god. Instead, he was a teacher who shared his wisdom based on his own discernment and experiences in life. This lack of an invisible deity often speaks to those that cannot find solace or belief in other religions where God is their governing body. Though there are many tales and teachings in Buddhism, there is no one holy book such as a Bible or Quran. Instead, the "bible" of Buddhism can be found in every natural effect on the planet, from the leaves on the trees to the worms in the ground. They are the story of the past, but you don't need to look to the past to find enlightenment, you need to look at every moment that you experience.

Moreover, the belief system of Buddhism is one that can be described as "large-minded." This means that those who practice it are open to accepting the moral teachings of other belief systems. Therefore, they are unconcerned with labels that pertain to specific religions, such as "Catholic," "Baptist," "Hindu," "Muslim," or even "Buddhist" itself. It is not uncommon to find those of different religious background meditating together at various Buddhist centers, especially in the western world. Enlightenment, in Buddhism, is not based on who you believe created you, but rather by opening your mind enough to allow yourself to shine through. Once that is reached, all the answers you seek on creation will be known to you. Therefore, your title of faith is of no concern, though, those who strive for enlightenment do usually find themselves identifying as Buddhist or other similar namesakes.

Buddhists neither seek an expansion of an organization nor attempt to convince others of a certain belief. Instead, they only provide an explanation if asked. The Buddha encourages one to be curious through awareness; therefore, Buddhism can be regarded more as a way of life-based on discernment rather than faith.

Though Buddhism as a practice can bend and move on a scale depending on your dedication to the teachings and heritage, anyone can practice the Buddhist way of living. There is always an extreme importance put on the word empathy, throughout the teachings of Buddhas through the generations. Empathy is not just reserved for humans, but for every living creature of this world.

At this point, you must be eager to learn the different teachings of the Buddha. Keep in mind that the Buddha's teachings are vast to such an extent that it grew into many different types of Buddhism. These teachings can bring wisdom to anyone, whether seeking to find their true self through enlightenment, or those that just wish to understand the world around them a little bit better. These teachings are for the young and old alike, regardless of religion, status, gender, or heritage.

However, let us not get ahead of ourselves.Before you do turn the page, though, please do remember the advice of the Buddha himself. It is to take care not to take his word for it but to test for yourself his teachings. Only by doing so will you then be able to find the true meaning of his words.

You have to discern the truth for yourself because your

truth will not be everyone else's. With the constant changes that happen throughout life, the Buddhist belief encourages that you embrace the moment and are ever present in it. For westerners, this is always a little difficult, since we are always striving to better ourselves, although sometimes the betterment that we seek is actually detrimental. Boasting is not part of the Buddhist way of life which is in contrast to the life in a modern society which encourages competition and heroics that have very little to do with betterment from a Buddhist point of view.

Chapter 3.
The History of Buddhism

You need to learn more about Buddha and Buddhism before you can delve into the Buddhist way of life and find your means to free yourself from stress and anxiety. You can start by learning about Buddha's origins and understand the reasons behind his way of life.

Siddhartha Gautama is the original name behind the famous man we know as Buddha. Gautama was born at the foothills of the Himalayan mountains around 567 BC in a place called Lumbini. Lumbini is known as Rummindei today and is situated close to Kapilbastu, which is on the northern edge of the Ganges River basin, southern Nepal. He was born during the late Vedic Period, which was in force between 800 and 500 BC in India. The Vedic period was a male-controlled Indian cultural period of time where individual people's membership was dependent on their father's ancestry. The Indian tribes were situated on the border of the Ganges River Valley at the time of Gautama's childhood.

The people in this valley were divided into tribal republics and were ruled by an elected leader or council of elders. It's historically unclear how these tribal groups were incorporated into the Ganges River Basin caste. A caste is a social order of people. There were 16 city-states in the central Ganges Basin and these were ruled by kings who were often at war with each other. Gautama's family belonged to the Kshatriya warrior caste.

The rise of these Indian cities and their courts brought social, political, and economical changes. These changes are often thought to have contributed to the ways of Buddhism. Buddhist texts mention various teachers who taught meditation, yoga, and asceticism to groups of followers, they followed a philosophical way of life. An ascetic person is someone who denies physical and psychological desires to attain a spiritual ideal or goal. These teachers focused on the nature of people and the consequences of their actions. Even though Buddha became a similar teacher of these ideas, he was still considered unique (Lopez, n.d.).

Gautama was an intelligent young man growing up. He was tall, strong, and handsome. Gautama's mother is known as Maha Maya and the Indian Brahmins prophesied Gautama's birth 12 years before he was born. They told of Gautama being a universal monarch or a great mentor. A Brahmin is another name for Indian priests or teachers.

Gautama's family were wealthy royals and his father kept him in the confines of their palace to prevent him from becoming a philosopher. Gautama grew up in a luxurious world as a young prince. He was protected from the outside world by his royal family and supplied with 500 attractive young women to entertain him through dance. His family also used sport to distract him, and he was trained by Brahmins in archery, swimming, wrestling, swordsmanship, and running. Gautama did exceptionally well in combat training and won himself a wife with his archery skills. His wife's name was Yasodhara, and she gave Gautama a son. Some people say that Gautama had everything.

Gautama didn't believe that he had everything and had a strong yearning to go beyond the palace walls. Gautama couldn't bear his curiosity anymore, and when he was 29-years old, he convinced his father to allow him to journey beyond the walls. He encountered three people in the streets of Kapilavastu on his exploratory visit that would change his life forever.

The people who changed Gautama was a sick man, an old man, and a dead man. Sadly, the locals were carrying these people to the fire to burn them. Gautama had always lived an easy life and nothing could have prepared him for this horrid experience. It was after Gautama's chariot driver told him that all living things will become sick, old, or die eventually, Gautama understood that these tragedies would befall his loved ones too. Gautama couldn't accept this and found rest difficult thereafter.

Gautama came across an ascetic man on his return to the palace the next morning. The ascetic man was wearing a plain robe and deep in meditation. Gautama's eyes met with this man, and there was a moment where he could feel a mindful connection between them. It was at this moment that Gautama realized that the answers to the question of suffering were inside the mind and not outside the body.

Gautama knew he had to become mindful to find refuge and experience mindful freedom for himself. He said goodbye to his wife and child in the middle of the night without waking them and left his home. Gautama rode to the edge of the forest because he couldn't bring himself to ignore suffering any longer. He used his sword to cut his long hair and traded his fancy clothes for plain robes before entering the forest (Fields, 1997).

This would be the start of a historical journey for Gautama. Even Gautama could never have realized how his decision would have a compounding effect and be remembered for centuries to come.

How Siddhartha Gautama Became the Buddha

Gautama's secret getaway took him to the forest where he would spend the next six years trying to find enlightenment. Gautama used the words of many teachers to guide his journey to mindful freedom and master their techniques. He was accompanied by five ascetics and his determination to his cause was so strong that these men became his followers. Gautama spent much of the six years enduring pain, starving himself, and refusing to drink in order to find what he was looking for. He would double his efforts when he still never found answers.

Gautama couldn't reach the level of insight he sought until a young girl came along and gave him a bowl of rice. As he sat there with a bowl of rice, Gautama realized that physically punishing his body and self-denial were not the way to find what he was looking for. In fact, this was making his own suffering worse. He needed to change his approach if he wanted to find inner deliverance and spirituality. Gautama finished his bowl of rice, drank fresh river water and bathed in the river. Gautama's five ascetic followers believed that this was a sign that he had given up. These men didn't believe in earthly pleasures and the ways of the flesh, and they promptly left

Gautama after his renewed vision.

Gautama sat alone under the Bodhi tree in Bodhgaya that night and made a promise to himself. He would not leave this place until the truth he sought came to him. Gautama entered a deep state of meditation that lasted for six nights.

Suddenly, Gautama was faced with threats from Mara, an evil demon, who challenged his entitlement to become Buddha. Mara attempted to steal Gautama's enlightenment as his own and Gautama touched the ground beside him and asked the earth to bear witness to his enlightenment. The earth did so, and Mara was banished.

Gautama's mind opened to the universe at this moment and a picture started to form in his mind. All his mixed feelings and rigid ideas dissipated as he entered the present moment. There was no separation in time and space anymore and Gautama became timeless. He finally saw the answer to the question of suffering that he'd been seeking for so many years. This was the exact moment where Siddhartha Gautama became Gautama Buddha – the Awakened One. Some people call him the Shakyamuni Buddha.

Buddha's journey continued just over a 100 miles away. After Buddha left the Bodhi tree, he came across the five ascetic followers who had left him in the forest. The same five followers who had abandoned Buddha on the eve of his awakening. Buddha encouraged them to follow a path of balance rather than a path characterized by artistic radicalism or severe discipline. Buddha referred to this path as the Middle Way. He gave his first lesson to these men and a crowd who had gathered along with them. This had set in motion the wheel of the dharma. He continued to explain the Four Noble Truths and the Eightfold path which are the pillars of Buddhism today. I will discuss these pillars in greater detail later in the book.

The ascetics became his first disciples and created the foundation of the Sangha. The word "sangha" means a community of monks or awakened people. The Sangha allowed women to join and class, race, gender, and ancestry mattered no more. The desire to reach mindful freedom through cleansing yourself of suffering and spiritual emptiness were the only considerations.

Buddha journeyed on foot through northern India and his journey continued for 45 years. He taught people from all castes, professions, and titles without discrimination. Kings and courtesans welcomed his teachings and Buddha answered all their questions with answers that were realistic. Buddha inspired his followers to question his teaching throughout his life and this remains prevalent in the Buddhist way of life today.

For the rest of Buddha's life, he continued to teach the Dharma. His ultimate goal was to lead others on the path of freedom to overcome their suffering. Gautama Buddha died at the age of 80 in 483 BC. Buddha told his disciples to follow no leaders but to be their own light and guide. On his deathbed, Buddha said, "I can die happily. I haven't kept a single teaching hidden in a closed hand. Everything that's useful, I have given. Now it's time to be your own guiding light." Buddha's followers began to teach his way of life after he died and this is how Buddhism was born. Gautama Buddha's way of life is called dharma (Buddha, 2015).

An important excerpt from this is that Gautama saw

suffering. He built his entire way of life around suffering and suffering includes stress, anxiety, depression, and negative thoughts. In addition, Gautama Buddha was young when he started his journey. In order to set the ball rolling, you should change your way of life while you're young.

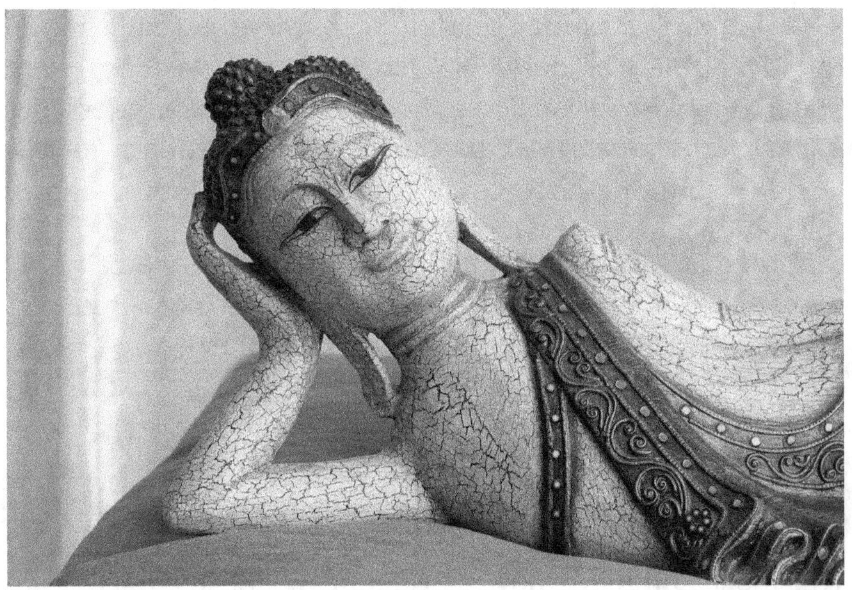

Photo: Reclining Buddha sculpture

Is Buddhism a Religion or Philosophy?

In order to use Buddhism to reach a place of inner peace within yourself and overcome all the stress and anxiety you suffer from, you need to see Buddhism as a way of life and not a religion.

This would make certain practices a religion. Results show that different Buddhist teachings will prove that it's in fact both a religion and a way of life. However, many followers of Buddhism don't recognize a higher god and instead focus on achieving freedom, wisdom, and inner peace for themselves. This is Buddhism's ultimate goal after all. So the choice lies with you whether you want to follow Buddhism religiously or as a way of life.

Enlightenment is also known as Nirvana. Nirvana is the mind's freedom from desires and its ability to live in peace. It's not an afterlife; it's only freedom from suffering and an understanding of it. Nirvana requires you to rid yourself of negativity such as lust, hatred, pain, anger, envy, and illusion. These are all insecurities that impact your stress levels. You'll never be reborn in this world of suffering once you have reached enlightenment.

Different Buddhist teachings believe that Nirvana can only be reached by monks and priests, but the main Buddhist philosophy teaches you that anyone can reach enlightenment. All the Buddhist teachings follow the words of Buddha who is identified as the great sage philosopher and not a god. Buddha never saw himself as a god or deity either but rather a teacher or a mentor.

The most common form of Buddhism doesn't encourage reincarnation because an individual tries to reach mindful freedom in a single lifetime. You're encouraged to be compassionate and understanding toward all living beings. I'll focus more on different teachings in detail later on.

Self-enlightenment is reached through meditation. It's meant to help you reach your own inner peace and understand your suffering on a whole new level. Some teachings encourage helping others attain enlightenment and some don't. Keep in mind, you're still subject to suffering, but you learn to overcome it and live with it.

Christians, Catholics, and Muslims don't recognize

Buddhism as a religion even though there are scriptures that date back farther than Jesus and Mohammed. Another reason for them to not recognize Buddhism as a religion is because of their belief in the word faith. According to the dictionary, the word faith is defined as believing in something or someone that has no evidence to back your belief. There's evidence of Buddhism and its success. These scriptures do however instruct you on a particular way of life.

In addition, there's no universal symbol for Buddhism. There are however a few images that have evolved and represent Buddhism. These include the lotus flower, the eight-spoked dharma wheel, the Bodhi tree, and the swastika. The Buddhist swastika means well-being or good fortune in Sanskrit.

Buddhism allows you to believe in learning from life experiences and is filled with structured practices. It's used worldwide on a daily basis to help non-followers learn to open their minds and help free themselves from stress, anxiety, and depression.

Buddha supplied us with a wide range of instructions and we can choose to follow the instructions to improve our own lives. You don't have to teach Buddhist philosophy to others. You can simply follow these instructions to overcome problems, become more compassionate and live a better life. This argument suggests that Buddhism is a way of life more than a religion (Essays UK, 2018).

Now that you understand the basics of Buddhism a little better, it's time to move on to understanding the different types of Buddhism that are common in the world today.

Chapter 4.
Teaching of Buddhism

Clearly, Buddhism has a long and rich history throughout the world. From Siddhartha Gautama's journey to enlightenment to the worldwide acceptance of Buddhism today, there is much to learn about this way of life. In this beginner's guide, the goal is to gain a broad overview of knowledge about Buddhism. Now that you understand more about how Buddhism came to be, it is time to learn about the basic principles, teachings, and philosophies practiced in Buddhism.

Dharma – The Path to Perfect Enlightenment

When the Buddha reached Nirvana, he did this by following the path of the dharma. In Buddhism, dharma refers to a sort of cosmic law and order – a way of thinking that believes there is a greater force at work than anything within us; not a divine god, but a divine force that ensures the scales are always balanced. Dharma is one of the 3 jewels of the Buddha, which we discuss later. The dharma can be thought of as the binding beliefs surrounding Buddhism – binding because when the dharma is realized and acknowledged, buddhas are created; the dharma binds the Buddhist community together under the umbrella of shared philosophies.

The dharma encompasses the entire path to perfect enlightenment, from your first moment of curiosity that leads you to explore Buddhism to the final moment when you achieve Nirvana. The Buddha said that the dharma is always here, always around us. The dharma is the foundation of our reality – it is who and what we are, it is the truth of who and what we are. Buddhists want to reach this "true nature," this "true self" that lies within. They do not want to just see it and recognize it; they want to relish in it, to live in it, and to forget any other self they might have been. Buddhists know that what we have no end and no beginning – it is an eternal circle of love. Everyone – even you – can follow the dharma, for this "true self" is within you, it is just on the edge of your consciousness. You only need to tap into it.

The dharma offers protection from all of the negativity around you. Buddhists believe that the problems and suffering we experience in our daily lives stems from ignorance. To eliminate ignorance, you simply have to follow the dharma. Dharma improves your quality of life. It does not focus on external factors, such as wealth and material objects, but rather, it focuses on improving your internal perception of your quality of life. True happiness comes from within, rooted firmly in your inner peace, tranquility, and joy. Buddhism teaches you that inner peace must come first; without it, there will never be peace on the outside. Inner peace is achieved through the spiritual paths of the dharma.

It is easiest to think of the dharma simply as the truth. It is your true self, your true reality, your true perception of life, your true peace, and your true happiness. The dharma teaches you how to grow mentally and intellectually – it is an expansion of your mind and your spiritual self, an expansion that reaches a level of pure bliss and peace – Nirvana. The dharma is much more than just a belief – it is a way of living your life. In fact, Buddha's teachings instructed his students to release all beliefs and speculations that they might hold.

The Buddha never took a stand on other's speculation and beliefs. He did not criticize other beliefs; rather, instead of offering some sort of judgment against other speculations and beliefs, he simply said that doing so:

"Is not beneficial, does not belong to the basics of the holy life, does not lead to disenchantment, to dispassion, to cessation, to peace, to direct knowledge, to enlightenment, to Nirvana."

—Middle Length Discourse 63.8

The Buddha taught the dharma as a way of life, a way to end suffering, as an actual practice that you can incorporate into your everyday life to reach Nirvana. The dharma is a way to live your life. The dharma is the practice of doing no evil and purifying your mind. There are no scriptures to memorize, no commandments to follow. Instead, the dharma focuses on the actions you take in life, the way you conduct yourself in life, and the moral principles by which you should live your life. These actions include things such as not criticizing others, not hurting others, knowing and practicing moderation, understanding solitude and how it opens your mind, and to always pursue a higher and more open state of mind. The dharma not only focuses on how you live your life through moral actions, but also expanding your mind, for without the expansion of your mind to a higher level of spiritual awareness, you will never reach Nirvana, and you will never end your suffering.

The dharma is your path to being indifferent, to being unencumbered, to simplify your life and belongings, to being modest, to being content, to being independent, to being persistent in your actions and goals, and to being completely unburdened. The dharma are the Buddha's teachings, the morals, and actions that he lived by. You, too, can live by the dharma, so you can live this same peaceful, unburdened, untroubled life of simplicity and happiness. The Buddha wanted only for people to live without arguing and fighting amongst each other. He created the dharma as a sort of roadmap for people to follow, a map that leads you to a life free from the worrying, suffering, and problems that plague your life. For with the right perception of the world around you, with an enlightened state of being, the worrying, problems, and suffering no longer matter – you find your peace.

The dharma teaches you that you must first see all of the negativity in your mind before you can let go of the negativity, and live a life of peace and happiness. You have to recognize within yourself and your own mind things such as anger, hate, greed, envy, and arrogance. Once you recognize and acknowledge all of the negativity in your mind, you are free to abandon it. You consciously leave it behind, choosing to know the dharma, to live a life of peace and happiness. Imagine the liberation, the freedom, that you can experience by leaving all of the negativity behind. This includes negative thoughts and feelings, as well as actions. Negativity has an energy all its own – it seeps into your life in all of the cracks, and it takes up residence within your mind. By learning to let go, you will no longer feel the overwhelming pressure of negativity.

The dharma is within all of us; it lies dormant within every mind, body, and soul. It is the path to Nirvana, which the Buddha defined as "the destruction of greed, hatred, and delusion." You see, each individual has the dharma inside of them, it is within their reach; they only have to see it. Each person can let go of the greed, anger, hatred, and delusion within themselves, and they can live a life of peace and harmony. Imagine what kind of world we would live in if ALL people found their dharma, letting go of all of the negativity, and living in peace and happiness? You can, too, know the dharma; it dwells within you, just out of sight and out of reach. All you have to do is see it within your mind and heart, and you will achieve Nirvana.

The Noble Eightfold Path

The Noble Eightfold Path is one of the primary teachings of the Buddha. The Noble Eightfold Path is visually represented by the Buddhist symbol of the dharma wheel. The dharma wheel is one of the oldest Buddhist symbols. It is believed that the Buddha set the wheel into motion upon the delivery of his first sermon teaching about Buddhism. The wheel is a symbol of the cosmic order of things, which we know is part of the dharma – a cosmic law and order. A wheel is always in motion, always moving; hence, it symbolizes the constant movement of the cosmic order of life.

You will remember that Buddhism is the philosophy of seeking liberation from the suffering of life. The Noble Eightfold Path is a sort of guide to show you how to end the suffering that comes with every life. Almost the entire philosophy of Buddhism draws from this path. Its very essence is found within so many of the Buddha's teachings, so many of his beliefs that he spread to his disciples, and then they spread throughout the world. The 8 practices of the Noble Eightfold Path are as follows:

Right understanding – understanding the way things really are, understanding the truth of things, knowing that every action has a consequence. This practice teaches you how to truly understand the world around you, a deep understanding that only comes with a pure and developed mind.

Right thought – knowingly giving up your material home and taking on the life of simplicity, modesty, love, and kindness, extending your thoughts of love and kindness to every living creature. This practice teaches you about releasing the bad while retaining the good. It teaches you to spread the goodness to everyone you come across in life.

Right speech – never lie, never gossip or slander another in a way that brings hatred and disharmony, never speak ill, rudely, maliciously, or abusively of another person. This practice teaches you to use kind, gentle, friendly, and useful words, words that have meaning, words that have the truth. If you cannot say something useful, keep a "noble silence."

Right action – never kill or injure another, never steal, give up material things, give up illegitimate sexual acts. This practice teaches you to conduct yourself in a moral, peaceful manner, with honor. It also teaches you to lead by example, to show others how to conduct themselves in the same honorable manner.

Right livelihood – only have just enough to live, to sustain a living, never work in a trade that harm's another living creature. This practice teaches you how to live with just enough so that you made abandon greed and envy. It also reinforces war and other professions that bring with them evil and harm to others.

Right effort – letting go of the negative, embracing the positive, ridding yourself and others of evil, creating positive, good, and wholesome states of the mind. This practice teaches you to, essentially, let go of the bad while holding on to the good. It also encourages you to show others how to eliminate evil from their lives.

Right mindfulness – always mindful of the Buddhist teachings, always conscious of your actions, always aware of your feelings, your thoughts, and your ideas. This practice teaches you to always know what is going on within yourself, as well as to give careful thought to your actions. This goes hand-in-hand with letting go of the negativity and embracing the good in life. It teaches you to be always conscious and aware at every moment so that you will always put forth kindness, love, and happiness.

Right concentration – practice meditation, develop your mindfulness, train and discipline your mind. This practice teaches you the stages of meditation. This first stage is when you discard all unwholesome thoughts from your mind, feeling only joy. The second stage is when you, essentially, clear your mind of any mental activities, teaching it to become still and tranquil, while you still feel the happiness and joy. The third stage teaches you to let go of the joy while still remaining happy. The fourth stage of meditation is when you release even the feelings of happiness, when your mind is a pure place, feeling and thinking nothing, only being aware.

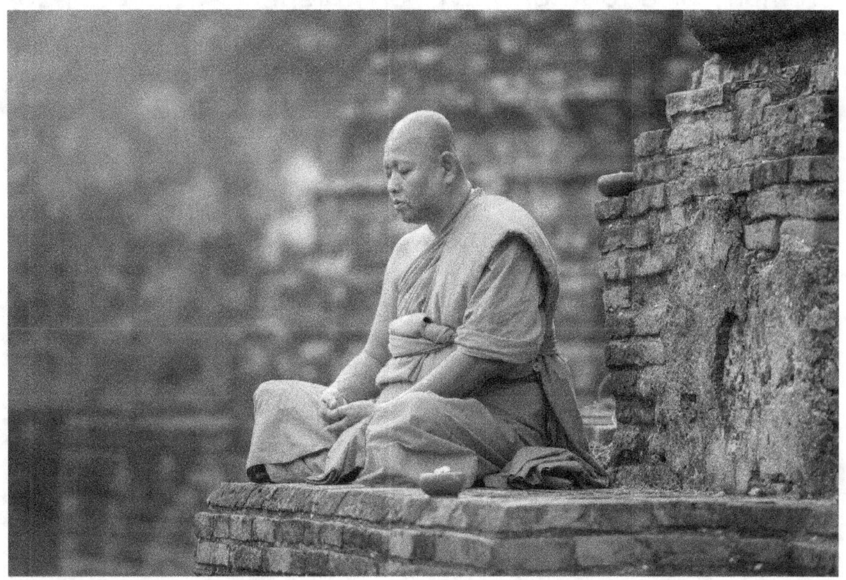

Photo: Buddhist monk

There is no right or wrong numerical order in which to follow the practices of the Noble Eightfold Path. The list is just that – a list of the practices. The primary goal of a burgeoning Buddhist is to develop each practice at the same time. Each practice builds upon other practices. As a Buddhist, you must work to develop the practices within yourself as far as you are capable of doing. Each practice is going to take time to nurture and develop. Do not expect immediate results – the path of Buddhism is a long one, one that is full of many, many steps.

The Eightfold Path is a path that is followed, practiced, and developed within yourself. Your path is not going to be the same as your fellow Buddhist's path. Each path is individual, each practice developed at your own pace, within your own skills. The Eightfold Path teaches you self-discipline, self-development, and self-purification. It is not a religious path upon which you will participate in a ceremony or a form of prayer or worship. This is the path of the Buddha, the very one that he followed, to reach freedom, peace, and perfect happiness – to reach Nirvana.

Chapter 5.
Karma and Rebirth

Buddhism is a non-theistic religion that focuses more on karma and not on any particular God. Karma is a word that is used today, but originated from the Hindu and Buddhist literatures. Not too many people in western society realize the origins of the word "karma," even though so many people use that word. Westerners think it means someone's fate or some spiritual system of justice that punishes bad people. This is not how the Buddhists define karma. Instead, Buddhists define karma as a willful action. In other words, every action you make will cause a similar action to be made towards you. Often times, people will think karma is the result of something. For example, if you cheat on a test, then the karma might be that you get caught and punished. This is not how the Buddhists view karma. They focus more on people who repeat their actions and then end up in a bad situation. In the same example, let's say you didn't get caught cheating on the test. Karma would dictate that you will likely cheat again in the future because people have a tendency of repeating their actions. As they keep repeating them, they are going to end up in a bad situation in the future. That is the true Buddhist way of viewing karma.

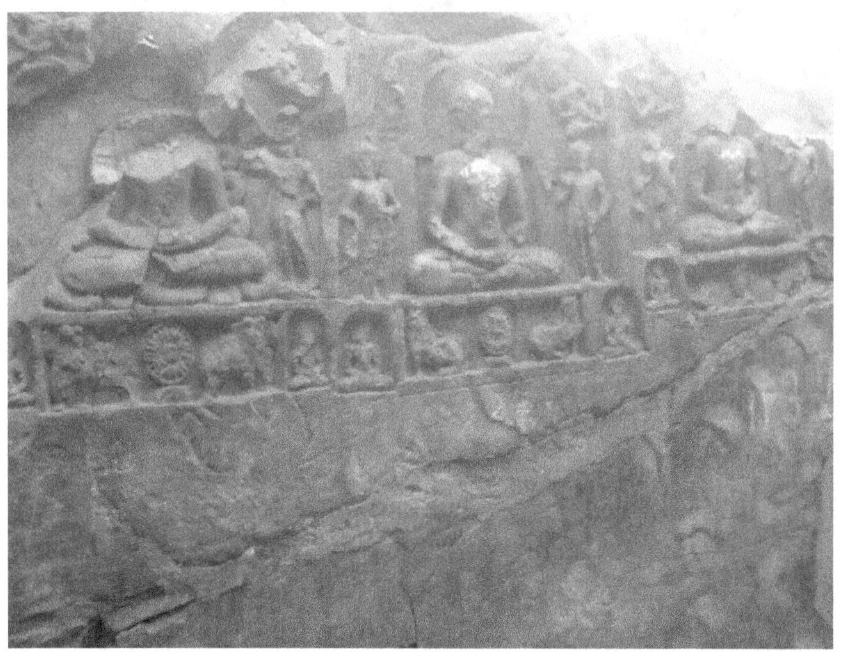

Photo: Ancient cave in India depicting Buddha meditating

Buddhists teach that in order to make a positive change in our lives, it requires us to change our karma. In other words, we have to take a different course of action then the repeated action we keep on taking. For example, if someone is in an abusive relationship and keeps forgiving their partner for the abuse, their karma is going to cause them pain in the future because they keep forgiving their partner. However, if they change their karma by dumping their partner, then the abuse will stop and they will be happy again. It is about changing one's action for the better. Buddhism also tells us that there are other natural forces out there, besides karma, which helps shape our lives for the better or worse. These could be natural disasters, like hurricanes, that creep up and destroy our homes, or maybe even kill us. This doesn't happen because we were bad in our lives. It is just an unfortunate situation caused by a greater force outside of the realm of karma.

Karma is often associated with the Buddhist belief of rebirth. There are three karmas associated with this; mind, speech and body. For example, when you were alive, did you say kind things to other people? Did you work hard in order to care for others and do good deeds? Did you help educate people and stop them from inflicting suffering upon others? If you did all of these things, then your karma is excellent and you will have a great life after your rebirth. On the flip side, if you were rude and violent towards others then you will have a painful life next time. Again, don't think of this as a result of your lifestyle. The actions are what lead you towards a particular path in the afterlife. Remember though that Buddhists do not believe in thinking of themselves as physical beings or people. There is no "me' in Buddhism. There are only the actions that we take which make good and bad things happen. Everything from suffering, pleasure and peace of mind all come from taking a particular type of action. Karma represents the action that you take, not the fate that is in store for you. After all, you have the power to change your fate by changing your action.

Buddhists do not believe death is the final end to someone's life. They believe when you die, your soul gets reborn into a new life. As you may know, Buddhists believe that change happens all the time. This applies to our souls as well. According to Buddhist teachings, nobody has just one constant soul that stays with them throughout eternity. Our souls can change the same way our lives change. After our soul changes, it carries forward into our next life and that will determine the kind of life we live.

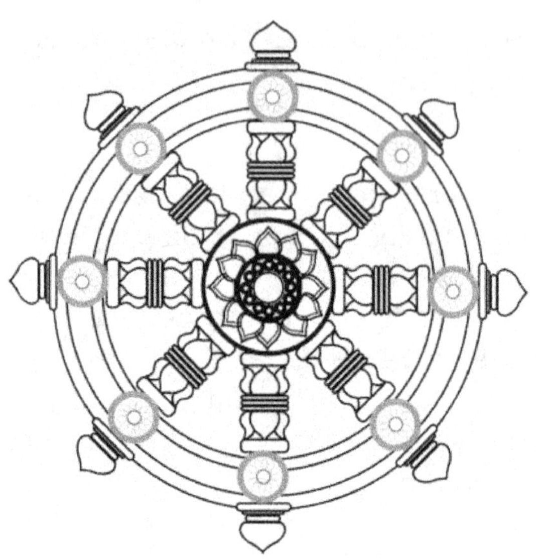

The wheel of life or continuous movement

Souls go through something called the "Wheel of Life." This wheel symbolizes samsara, which is a Buddhist word that means "continuous movement." Basically, when we die our soul moves through the wheel of life before we are reborn again. The wheel contains six possible paths that our soul can go through, which is what will change our soul. The paths are labeled as Godly, humans, demi-God, animals, hungry ghosts and hell-beings. The first three paths are where people who do good deeds go. Remember that Buddhism teaches people how to end suffering and what to truly value in life. If you go around helping other people, being friendly, and not caring about wealth or possessions, then chances are you will end up on one of the good paths. Basically, you have to refrain from the three poisons of Buddhism; stupidity, greed and hatred. So, if you are someone who has hurt people and caused suffering from your own greed then you will end up on one of the darker three paths.

When we get reborn from the path our soul has entered, our new life will endure the same feelings as the label we've been given. This means our next life will endure the same fears and sufferings that animals go through. After all, wild animals suffer all the time from being attacked by other predators or even eaten by them. Have you ever walked in the woods and come across a squirrel? What is the first thing the squirrel does when you go near it? The squirrel runs away quickly or climbs up a tree at rapid speed. It does this because it is always in fear that something is going to attack it. These are the feelings that someone born through the animal path will end up feeling in their next life. As for the other paths, the hungry ghost is someone who is constantly hungry and thirsty. They spend their lives looking for food and being frustrated. The hell path is the worst. It inflicts at least 18 different types of torment upon a person, including excessive coldness, hotness, deformities, disabilities and more.

The good paths are pretty diverse, but they are definitely where you want to be. The human path is not as radiant as the other two good paths, but it is the only path that allows you to practice dharma. These are the disciples and followers of Buddhism who teach the religion to other people. Unfortunately, they will be subjected to the risks of pain and suffering, but they can also get pleasure as well. As for the demi-God path, you will have an abundance of pleasure but you will also be fighting a lot of wars and battles. Now the best path you can end up in is the Godly path. These people live the longest and most joyous lives possible. They don't practice dharma and they don't fight wars. They just live their lives in total happiness with very few moments of pain. However, when they eventually get out of this life they will end up back on one of the bad paths because they would have used up all of their good karma.

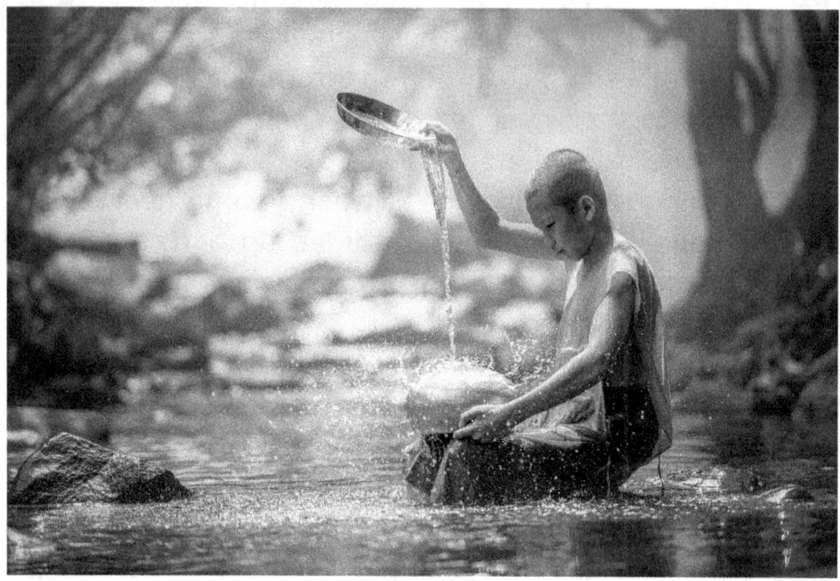

Photo: Water Ritual

Chapter 6.
Reincarnation

Some people believe that upon death, we disappear altogether: we simply return to the dust. This is a form of nihilism.

In contrast, others believe that our soul's existence is permanent: for example, they may believe that after death they can go up to the heavens and enjoy heavenly blessings forever, which is a common form of eternalism. Generally, eternalism is the belief that the self or soul has a fixed and essential nature that is eternal and cannot be destroyed.

In Buddhism, we take the Middle Way, and believe that our soul neither disappears entirely, nor exists permanently unchanged – rather, each soul cycles through reincarnation. We go through countless births and deaths as a result of our karma.

Reincarnation comes from the Sanskrit term samsara. Samsara is often translated as the "reincarnation wheel." A wheel usually embodies circular as well as vertical motion. The image of a wheel symbolizes how all living beings are born into various locations in the universe, and go through the various planes of existence non-stop – some high, some low, just like a wheel. It also symbolizes the fundamental, unbroken chain of cause and effect that dictates what types of bodies we will obtain each time we go through birth and death.

Everything in the universe goes through cycles of change. The evolution of living beings through the cycle of reincarnation is a dynamic process much like the changes that occur in the natural world around us.

Consider the four great elements of earth, water, wind, and fire which pass through natural changes in their states of being.

Take the element of earth. Originally, it is simply dirt. Then the potter molds it and bakes it into a vessel. Over time, the vessel gets destroyed and thus eventually returns to its original state of dirt.

Water has its own cycles, beginning with evaporation from the oceans and lakes. Vapor then ascends to the skies, where it is cooled and condenses into clouds. Clouds gather and eventually the water falls to earth as rain, returning to the original state of a liquid. And then the cycle begins again.

The wind element is just movement of air. Air is heated by the sun, expands and ascends to the skies, creating empty space. The low pressure of empty space causes air from other areas to be moved toward it, thus causing wind. The air movement can be slow or fast, creating gentle wind or violent tornadoes.

The great fire element originates from heat. When

conditions allow, heat can create fire. Potential heat already exists in all things and waits for conditions to manifest itself in the form of fire. For example, two wood sticks already contain heat in the form of energy stored in their molecular structure. When we rub them together, heat will manifest and create fire. In other words, fire also cycles through various states of manifestation, which may be visible or invisible to our eyes.

Our bodies are the result of the temporary union of these four great elements. For example, the great earth element gives our body solidity in the form of bones, muscles etc. The great water element constitutes our blood, tears etc. Our breathing and rhythms of the heart are based on the great wind element. Finally, our body heat is derived from the great fire element. Like the four constituent elements, our body must also go through reincarnation as driven by the forces of karma.

On a larger scale, each galaxy, which in Buddhism is known as a world, must also cycle through a kind of reincarnation. Each world must go through the four cycles of formation, dwelling, decay and emptiness. More specifically, each world first comes into existence, then reaches maturity, deteriorates, and finally disappears. Throughout the universe, one world comes into existence while others disappear in a wonderful cadence that is dictated by the laws of cause and effect.

Ordinary living beings cycle through the following six planes of existence as driven by the karma they have created:

The hell realms: Yes, the hells do exist. These are the last places that you want to be in.

The hells are characterized by extreme suffering. The prisoners there undergo constant torture through very lengthy terms. At the end of such terms, they tend to be reborn into the hells to continue undergoing their retribution.

How do we fall to the hells? If in this life, we plant the causes for going to the hells, then after our death, we will most likely be reborn there. In particular, succumbing to anger creates the seeds for falling into the hells.

The hungry ghosts' realm: Buddhism teaches that there are ghosts and spirits just as there are humans. Ghosts are predominantly yin beings; yin is the dark force that opposes yang in traditional Chinese philosophy and medicine. These beings are in great suffering because they are constantly thirsty and hungry. You have no idea what it is like until you have no water to drink or food to eat. It feels so bad that you want to die but you can't! Ghosts exist in the midst of our human world. However, we cannot usually see them because they are outside the range of our everyday perceptions, just like infrared light or radio waves, which exist at wavelengths that we cannot perceive.

How do we become hungry ghosts? If we harbor a greedy mind, we will plant the causes for receiving a hungry ghost body in the future.

The animal realm: The animal, ghost, and hell realms are together commonly referred to as the "three evil paths," because there is a lot of suffering there, the terms are very long and it is very hard to escape these realms.

How do we obtain an animal body? By planting the causes of stupidity. Just indulge in excessive sensual pleasures, live senselessly, surrender to your ego and you will definitely fall to this realm.

The asura realm: Asuras are present both in their own realm, which is a separate plane of existence from ours, and in all the other realms as well. Asuras are fond of fighting, arguing, and conflict for its own sake. For example, many asuras in our human realm become soldiers, boxers, or anyone with a combative nature. Even many established and respected professionals are asuras. You can recognize their asura nature immediately because they often contradict those around them, and insist on offering their opinion, even if unsolicited.

The Buddha predicted that after his death, the world would gradually decline. We see a pattern of conflict in our world today, and disharmony among cultures, religions, political groups and even youth. Few people devote their lives to practicing virtue, and many prefer, instead, to fight. Asuras are common in today's world.

The human realm: Humans are a mixture of yin and yang, a combination of goodness and evil. The human realm, as well as the subsequent heavenly realms, are much more conducive to cultivation than the other four types of rebirth.

In order to obtain a human body, we should cultivate the Five Precepts.

The heavenly realms: You plant the causes for birth to the heavens by cultivating the Ten Good Deeds and observing the Five Precepts.

In the heavens, everything is as you wish. You are reborn in the heavens because you have earned enough blessings that now you can sit back and enjoy them. The heavens are very blissful. The only drawback is that it is not a permanent solution. In time, those in the heavens will use up all of their blessings and fall back down to lower realms again, and the cycles of rebirth will continue.

These are the six common realms. In order to get out of the cycle of reincarnation, one must cultivate diligently to make it to the four sagely realms of the Arhats, Pratyekabuddhas, Bodhisattvas and Buddhas.

But first, let us look at some of the evidence in support of reincarnation.

There was a noted doctor who became a believer in reincarnation after one of his patients recalled past life traumas that assisted in relieving the anxieties and phobias she was experiencing in her life. His belief strengthened after seeing many more patients regress to past lives.

This doctor, who graduated from Columbia University and Yale Medical School, used both traditional therapy and hypnosis to help his patient overcome her symptoms. During hypnotic states, she experienced a series of past lives, and was able to speak to higher beings in an "in-between lives" state.

In addition, during a hypnotic state, the patient connected with the doctor's dead father and son, and related to to doctor that his son had died in infancy due to a rare heart condition. This was information she could not have known and the doctor became convinced his patient had tapped into another realm.

Here are some other stories of reincarnation.

In the first half of the 20th century in Delhi, India, lived an 8-year old girl named Phatedevin. She often cried and begged her parents to allow her to go to Mita, another city that was 120 miles away, so that she could see her husband. Perplexed, her parents asked a journalist to investigate the matter.

Phatedevin told the reporter that, in her past life, she had been married to a teacher and bore him a son. When their son was 11 years old, she fell sick and passed away. When the reporter pressed her for proof, she said that she buried gold, silver and jewels at specific locations. She also told him about a gift of a fan that bore some specific writings and was given to her by a friend.

He also verified everything the girl had claimed including the existence of the fan with the writings.

The reporter returned to Delhi and brought the girl and her parents back to Mita. Even though she had never left Delhi before, she was able to navigate the city streets of Mita and led them to the teacher's house.

As they entered the house, they met with an 80-year old man with white hair. The young girl was very happy and indicated that he had been her father-in-law.

This was reported in the major newspapers in India and many more newspapers in the world.

Sutton died in childbirth, leaving behind eight children.

As a young girl, Jenny spoke of her life in Ireland, and even drew a map of the small village where she was born; she could also describe the room where she had died in 1936..

After her death as Mary Sutton, her children had been sent to orphanages. As an adult, in her current life, Cockell was able to obtain six of her children's names with the help of a priest from an orphanage in Ireland.

In 1993, Cockell was able to track down her five surviving children and reunite with them during the filming of an Irish documentary about her journey. Cockell wrote a book about her story called "Across Time and Death." The story was dramatized in a CBS movie made for television in 2000.

The final incident we will refer to is a rather atypical occurrence of rebirth where one person's consciousness was reborn, not into the body of a newborn baby, but into another adult. It occurred in Ca Mau, Vietnam, in the prior century, where a girl fell ill and died at the age of 19 in the small village of Dam Gioi. At another village of Vinh My (Bac Lieu), there was at the same time a girl who was sick, but recovered. After she recovered, she no longer recognized her parents and behaved strangely. Her parents initially thought that this was probably due to side effects from her illness. When fully recovered, she started crying and insisted on getting permission to return to the village of Dam Gioi which she could describe in minute detail.

Her parents contacted the people of the Dam Gioi village and came across the family of the young girl who had died in Dam Gioi; they invited the family to come for a visit. As soon as they arrived in Vinh My, the daughter recognized the visitors as her own parents and shared family secrets that no one else could know. Eventually, she was recognized by both families and inherited their fortunes.

This was widely circulated in Vietnamese newspapers.

Some may be skeptical about the reality of reincarnation. But try to keep an open mind to the possibility that our consciousness has been migrating from body to body for a long time, propelled by causal forces that we created in the past.

If we have faith that reincarnation is real, then we would be wise to refrain from creating offenses in order to avoid falling to the lower realms, because once we have fallen, there is a lot of suffering and it is extremely difficult to extricate ourselves.

Further, we should make the effort to do good deeds in order to plant the causes for ascension so that we can one day escape the cycle of suffering and attain bliss – a central aim for the Buddhist cultivator.

Chapter 7.
The practice of Buddhism

Due to the practical nature of Buddhism and the way deities are looked upon, there's been an ongoing debate on whether it is, in fact, a religion. By definition, a religion has to be constituted of certain rituals and practices. Therefore, rituals are what make Buddhism a religion. It is possible to practice the Buddhist rituals and values without accepting any of the beliefs (unlike most other religions). This makes Buddhism a more secular and pragmatic religion focused on inner growth. The un-ordained practitioner (Buddhist layman/laywoman) will find it relatively easy to carry out the practices in his/her daily life.

Buddhism stems from the teachings of the Buddha focused towards a more wholesome life. Along with his teachings, he established a monastic and secular way of life with rules and guidelines for both paths (spiritual and material).

His teachings were very resourceful and gathered a large following. They spread across a vast region and incorporated a lot of cultural, historical and religious background from the native countries.

The different cultures that embraced Buddhism incorporated some of their rituals and practices into it. They blended the compatible customs of their own societies into Buddhism. This resulted in a religion rich with rituals and practices. Some of the fundamental rituals for all Buddhist paths are the following.

Meditation involves the practice of the mind.

Mantras are recitations of prayers and teachings.

Mudras involve hand gestures facilitating the subtle energies within.

Prayer Wheels are cylindrical wheels containing teachings or mantras.

Pilgrimage is a visit to sacred sites.

Seeking refuge means going to monasteries and focusing on one's practice.

Prayer is a seeking for blessings or fulfillment of aspirations.

Auspicious ceremonies accompany taking up Buddhist vow's or ordination, marriage, housewarming events or blessings for a new office.

Inauspicious ceremonies are related to someone passing away.

Daily rituals involve confessions, making offerings, a dedication of merit and paying homage.

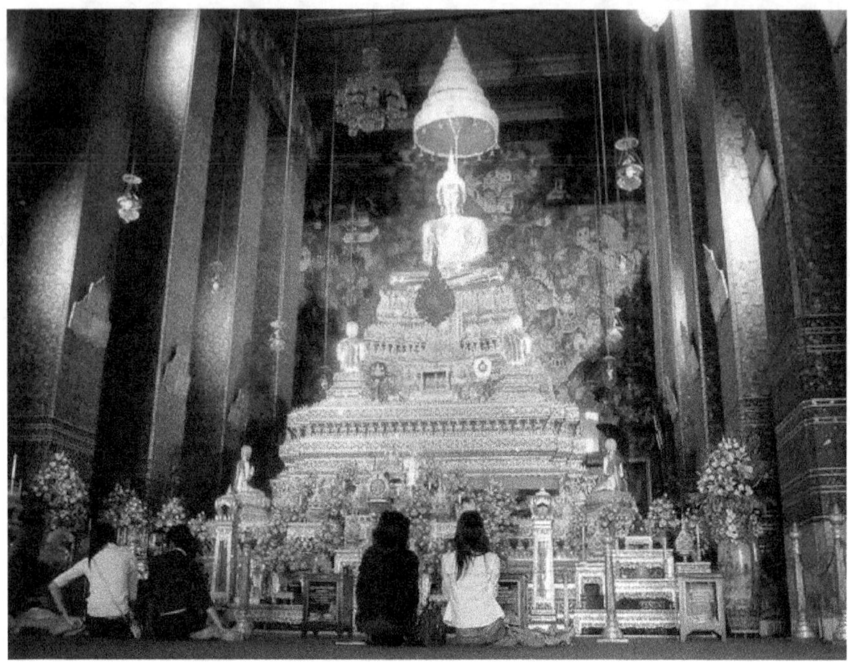

In general, the dedication of merit can accompany all aforementioned rituals as it involves intent toward sharing one's blessings.

There are many facets of Buddhist meditation practice that are followed in different parts of the world to achieve different goals. But for the more beginner/intermediate learner, we will cover only the most significant concepts without much loss in the essence.

We live in a society that imposes uncertainty upon us. There are issues that our mind can't handle from an early age. This process continues into adulthood and soon our minds get too busy. A great deal of it involves the actions of the people around us which usually make us turn toward our primal instinct to protect us from discomfort and pain.

We start overthinking everything and we act out of anger, fear or try to escape our reality. Our perception of reality is sometimes distorted as a defense mechanism.

Next, we start thinking about our suffering. We may not realize it, but our suffering can't be solved by thinking. It is like sitting in your room and reading about surfing. No amount of reading can get you to feel the wave. And yet, we're not even aware of that. Getting caught up in our mind, we seek sensory pleasure and over stimulate our senses. Long term, that results in a lowering of awareness of the true nature of things around us. The obvious solution is to become more aware, or mindful.

A usual misconception when it comes to the Buddhist concept of impurity of the body is that the point is to develop an aversion to sensory pleasures. Being mindful of the aforementioned is a tool to free our minds of the addiction to sensory pleasures. When you are completely mindful of your body, the sensory pleasures cease to hold you prisoner.

By practicing mindfulness, you can reach more peaceful states of existence where you get to experience joy, depend less on physical realities that are sensory illusions etc. Mindfulness is a powerful weapon that we have to add to our arsenal against suffering. But how do we do that?

The first step is to focus on breathing. Breathing is quintessential to our existence. When we shift our focus to breathing, we start to practice mindfulness. We became aware of the all the thoughts that occupy our mind.

We are being more aware of our real environment and

the present moment. The next step in practicing mindfulness is letting go and to stop trying to fight those thoughts. By becoming less judgmental of ourselves and others, we decrease the power that our thoughts and emotions have over our actions.

Then we start to notice the positive aspects of reality that we wouldn't have seen if we were trapped by our undesired states of mind.

When we start cultivating mindfulness, we are easily able to distance ourselves from our thoughts. This gives us more capacity to deal with our issues. As we become more mindful of the present, our memory also improves.

With patience and mindfulness, we can come to the realization of the root cause of our problems. The practice of mindfulness can give us the energy to deal with those problems.

What comes next? When we develop our consciousness and awareness, we realize that other people are suffering too. Sometimes we might be able to help them. By shifting our focus from ourselves, our suffering which we might not be able to deal with at the present moment becomes less of a problem.

There are many ways to cultivate mindfulness. Breathing is the starting point. We can also practice mindfulness while walking. By focusing on every step and our breathing, we are essentially practicing walking meditation.

For mindfulness to develop into a habit, we need to practice it daily in conjunction with a routine (preferably in the morning). With a few simple triggers and routines (explained in the book linked above), we can easily turn mindfulness into a part of our lives. At that point, mindfulness becomes a quality of our character. It becomes a way of seeing things, a way of handling and dealing with reality.

Mindfulness lets us dwell a bit deeper into our consciousness as well. We become aware of all the superficial thoughts that are on autopilot. Vipassana takes this one step further.

Vipassana lets us use mindfulness and the awareness of our breath to calm ourselves to a point where we get in touch with our subconscious mind.

We can compare it to an ocean. The surface of the ocean has waves that are visible. As we go deeper into the ocean, there are not many waves to notice. Eventually we can't see the currents that are present but only feel their presence.

Vipassana is a great meditation practice for beginners. There are layers to it but the basic requirement is the determination to feel more at peace within you and act in a more wholesome manner.

The first step in Vipassana meditation is to choose a position where you will feel relaxed but will still be able to focus without falling asleep.

While choosing a sitting position, the most important part is for you to feel comfortable. If you're at ease sitting cross-legged, there are a few positions you may choose – the easy pose, a half lotus or a full lotus pose.

You might want to support your back with a pillow if you

experience any tension. If you're unable to sit down, you might consider sitting on a chair.

The easier pose is just sitting cross-legged; the half lotus is placing one foot on the upper thigh of the opposing leg while the full lotus requires both feet at the opposing thighs.

Another important facet to consider is the length of your meditation session. It is advised to prepare you and ease into it. For beginners, five minutes should be enough.

You can increase your meditation sessions over time. Keep in mind that Vipassana meditation is practice, but try to make it a pleasant experience, in the sense that you're not overly exerting yourself.

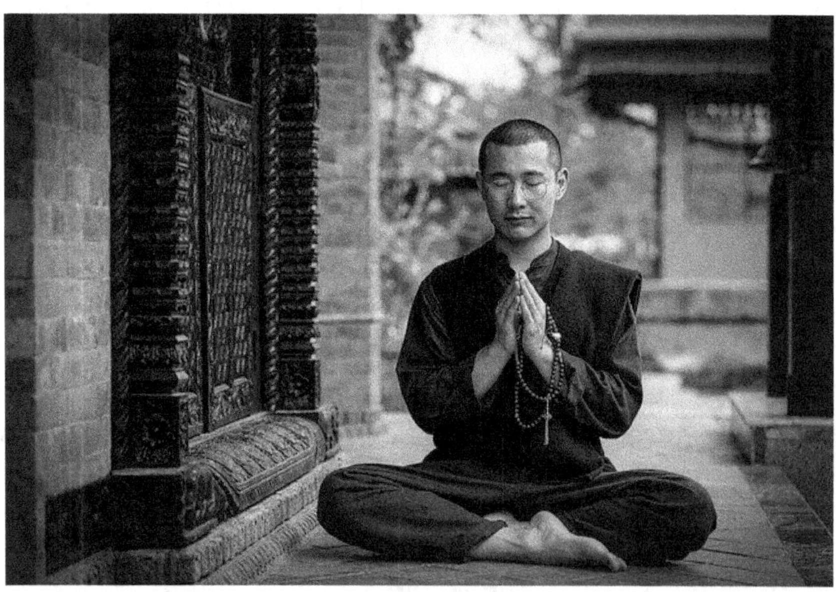

If you're serious about Vipassana meditation, you can increase your sessions up to one hour in the morning and another hour at night. In longer and deeper meditative states, you might experience a significant amount of discomfort. If you do, it is advised that you consult with a meditation expert at this point. This is when your mind is doing the heavy lifting and you need someone to help you lift the burden.

Vipassana meditation is referred to as 'thought watching meditation', so it can be referred to as mindfulness meditation as well. Every movement of the body comes from the mind. While sitting still, all of the subconscious thoughts and emotions will emerge at some point.

After assuming a comfortable position, try to sit as straight as it's comfortable and lengthen your neck and spine, with your chin lightly tucked towards the neck.

If you're feeling stiffness, just experience it and try to relax those muscles. Your body remembers when it had a straight posture and with practice, you can actually improve it.

Experience the thoughts, emotions, and images as they arise and let them go. Stay as detached from them and observe them as if they're not a part of you. Continue doing this as your train of thought goes on.

There will be moments when your mind goes blank. Use those moments to rest your mind. If you observe any affinity or dislike towards a thought or a reflection, let it go. When some particularly disturbing thought patterns or images appear, simply divert your attention towards your breath.

When you experience something unpleasant during Vipassana meditation that you're unsure how to get rid of, try taking a deep breath and try to release it as you exhale.

As you clear your mind, gently bring back your attention to the body and to the breath. Observe the tranquil moment and how you're feeling during it. When you're ready, slowly lift your head up and take in your surroundings. You've just experienced a session of Vipassana meditation.

Chapter 8.
Mindfulness Meditation Techniques and Self-Healing Meditation

"Meditation means the recognition or the discovery of one's own true self."

Sri Chinmoy

Meditation indeed helps you discover and understand yourself. For that to happen, you need to get started with the practice.

There exists countless meditation techniques created and improved on over the years. While all of them are amazing and effective, some of them are 'better' or 'kinder' to beginners.

The "Do Nothing" Meditation Technique

The sages of countless spiritual cultures and traditions believe that the highest state of intuition and spiritual awakening occurs in our minds and is present all the time.

This means 'enlightenment' has always been a part of your mind, is present even now, and will forever be there.

Hinduism refers to enlightenment as 'self,' while Buddhism calls it as the 'Buddha nature.' This means that true awakening is a part of your system and is present at all times. However, you need to trigger it, fuel it, and sustain it to keep it active at all times.

Since we are rarely aware of ourselves, rarely live in the present moment, and are normally functioning in the 'monkey or small state' of mind, our spiritual awakening lies dormant. For the 'awareness' light bulb to shine bright, we need to switch it on.

The 'Do Nothing' meditation technique does this quickly and effectively.

About the Technique

Zen Buddhism calls the 'Do nothing' technique "shikantaza," a term that translated means "just sitting." The Tibetan version of Buddhism calls it "dzogchen." Krishnamurti, the famous Hindu meditation teacher, called it "choice-less awareness."

The main idea behind this technique is that while total awakening is a part of your mind, you cannot notice it at all times. One obstruction that keeps us from switching on that awareness is the sense of being a 'doer.' In other words, doing things, what I call 'doership,' lies at the core of one's sense of self. We are always ready to do something and feel strange when there is nothing to do even though many of us yearn for some time to sit idle. However, even when we are 'idle,' we still engage ourselves in something meaningless.

When you let go of that need to put in effort, the sense of constantly trying something, and the tendency to choose to do something all the time, you diminish and relax your ego. To simplify it: the sense of making decisions and volition is actually the sense of one's self. This is not just a random theory. There is sufficient neuro-scientific research to prove it.

The human brain has a structure called the 'posterior cingulate cortex' (PCC) that serves as the main player in your default mode network (DMN.) This mode is active whenever you feel distracted or think about yourself. A study discovered that increased DMN activity produces negative emotions, which means preoccupation with one's self often makes us feel bad.

Functional magnetic resonance imaging (FMRI) brain scans illustrate that PCC activity tends to slow down when you let go of the constant need to do something. When you feel that everything around you is happening effortlessly, activity in your DMN and PCC start to slow down more, which helps you feel good, relaxed, and calmer.

In fact, when you let go of things and allow everything around you to unfold seamlessly, you allow things to flow easily and achieve the 'peak experience' state that happens only when something you have been doing for years becomes a part of your automatic response.

By practicing the 'Do nothing' meditation technique, you can easily (and quickly) activate the 'flow state,' a state that when consistently activated, switches on spiritual awakening in your mind.

How do you practice the "do nothing" meditation technique? Let us discuss that:

How to Practice "Do Nothing" Meditation

This is by far the easiest meditative technique anywhere in the world. This meditation technique requires you to do ABSOLUTELY NOTHING but just sit down, unwind, and switch on your sense of awareness.

Yes, that is it: relax, and sit somewhere (preferably) quiet without worrying about anything.

If you still can't get it, here is a step-by-step process to carry it out.

Find a nice, clean, and calm spot to relax and meditate in. It could be a corner of your house, your patio, your bedroom, or anywhere outside, preferably some place quiet and that is free from the distraction of moving things. However, some people find it easier to practice 'do nothing' meditation in a garden or park, and not their own home because indoors, they somehow keep thinking of the tasks lined for the day and cannot do nothing for 5 minutes.

If you think you will feel distracted or bored after a few minutes and have a lot to do that day, set a timer for 5 to 10 minutes so when it beeps, you know you have to get up; this will help you stop the need to keep glancing at your watch.

Next, close your eyes—or keep them open; whatever feels convenient—and relax.

Very gently, pull your attention away from all the thoughts running around in your mind to simply nothing at all.

Remind yourself of how you need to let go of everything

that bothers you, and even thoughts that do not bother you, and not actively think.

Just stay in the very moment and either relax yourself by observing the sensations in your body, one after another, or open your eyes and look around and witness everything from an accepting, nonjudgmental perspective.

Yes, even though you are not actively doing something, you are still doing something- you are simply witnessing the moment and the things, thoughts, emotions, and experiences it brings forth, and then letting go of that too.

Every time you feel 'getting caught up' in some thought, just let it go. If you feel an emotion bubbling inside and holding you hostage, let it go too. If you are struggling not to think, just relax, and let go of that worry too. If any sort of tightening sensation or anything else bothers you, let go of that as well. To let go of something, simply take a deep breath and imagine that worry moving out of your system leaving you feeling light and relaxed.

Just keep relaxing yourself witnessing every moment as you experience it and quietly observing everything inside and around you. You do not have to actively do or think anything; just witness everything as a silent observer devoid of any judgments, viewpoints, or beliefs.

Keep at it for 5 to 10 minutes in the start and as you progress, increase the duration of your meditation sessions.

When the timer beeps, open your eyes—if you had closed them—and gently bring your realization back to the world around you and allow yourself to experience that transition. You will notice a newfound peace inside you. With that, get back to your routine chores with the intention to complete your tasks consciously and mindfully.

This meditation technique is simultaneously simple and difficult. Not doing anything or thinking sounds very easy to do. However, we have become used to functioning in the monkey state of mind and worrying about what to do next that we can hardly stop ourselves from not thinking or doing anything.

When you complete a session or two of the technique, you realize how simple it can be to do nothing and just silently watch your thoughts, emotions, feelings, and everything else, and let go of it so you stop holding on to anything meaningless, as this only increases your inner burden.

Regular practice of this technique strengthens your ability to relax and do nothing when you ought to be doing nothing. This way, every time you lie down to rest or are taking a time-out from your work, you actually relax instead of incessantly worrying about the mistakes you made or the things awaiting your input. This regulates the production of alpha and theta waves, something which helps you relax and feel peaceful; it also improves your sense of focus.

In addition to working on this technique, here are some more amazing and easy-to-do meditative techniques you can gradually incorporate into your routine to make meditation a constant part of your life.

Breathing Meditation

Your breath is the essence of your existence; if you stop breathing, you stop living. Although the breath is very important, unfortunately, we often disregard it and take it for granted, especially because we know breathing is an involuntary action.

Because of our disregard of the breath, we suffer from scores of emotional and physical health related problems. Even research validates this and countless research studies show how shallow and rapid breathing is one of the reasons behind anxiety, stress, depression, heart problems, and other issues.

To live a better, more peaceful and more meaningful life, you need to work on improving your breathing because when you feel healthy, you automatically feel peaceful.

In addition, becoming aware of your breath and its power makes you more appreciative of this ability and this improves your emotional wellbeing. Moreover, being aware of your breathing makes you more focused on the present moment.

In this meditation technique, you use your breath to anchor yourself to the present, something which helps you become grounded and more focused on the moment that is. This improves your ability to nurture awareness and the big state of mind. One of the most effectual ways of accomplishing that is by practicing mindfulness based breathing meditation for as little as 2 minutes daily. If done consistently, your awareness levels gradually improve greatly.

How to practice breath awareness meditation

Here is how to practice breathing meditation:

Find somewhere that is distraction free then sit down and relax.

Set your timer to beep after 2 or 5 minutes, depending on how long you want to meditate.

Close your eyes—or keep them open—and then gently bring your awareness to your breath. If possible, practice 'doing nothing' meditation for a few minutes prior to mindfulness based breathing meditation; it will help clear your mind of unnecessary thoughts so that you can focus better on the practice.

Watch your breath for the entire 2 to 5 minutes and use it as the object of your focus in order to cultivate connectedness with the present moment.

Watching your breathing means closely and mindfully observing it and becoming aware of it as it enters, circulates, and then leaves your body. Do not attempt to deepen your breath; simply breathe as you usually do. Yes, deep breathing is important, but right now, the purpose of this technique is not to deepen your breath. The purpose is to make you aware of your breath. With time and consistency, your breath will become deep all by itself and you will notice a massive decrease in your anxiety and stress levels.

Inhale through your nose and watch how the in-breath makes you feel. See if you can pinpoint any sensation your body experiences as a result of your breathing i.e. the rising and falling of your belly, or anything of that sort. When it is time to exhale, do so through your mouth and once again, watch your out-breath, any sensations it produces and how it makes you feel generally.

As you meditate, your mind will—not may—wander off in thought. When this happens, remember to be patient and gentle with yourself. Instead of labeling thinking as a 'bad practice' or assuming you are incapable of meditating or doing anything right, understand that you are new to meditation and as such, since your awareness is not strong, wandering off in thought is bound to happen. Let go of this concern and refocus on your breath. Refocus on your breath every time your mind wanders off, and if it helps, count your breath to keep better track of it.

When the timer beeps, gently and slowly shift your focus from your breath to your environment and take time to open your eyes or become more focused on the world around you.

Engage in this practice daily so that you become better at it. Within weeks, you will notice yourself gently observing your breath many times during the day and your general observation and awareness levels improving thus allowing you to stay mindful of everything with greater acceptance.

Mindfulness Eating

Meditation is not just about leaving everything and taking deep breaths or observing a single thought at a time. Meditation is more about awareness and if you do everything with deep awareness, you are in a state of meditation at all times. That can happen if you nurture a habit of staying mindful at all times. Mindfulness-based eating is definitely a great way to get the hang of that habit.

Eating is something we do often, an activity that gives us great pleasure. Nonetheless, not many of us are truly aware of what we eat or how we eat. Have you ever felt hungry shortly after eating a big steak? Do you ever think about how the mint margarita you just had tasted even though you loved it while you were hurriedly sipping it?

Even though you know food will not automatically vanish from your plate, you eat as if it would: quickly stuffing your mouth with one bite after another and gobbling down a big meal in mere minutes. This is how most of us eat and this is what leads to obesity, health problems, and the general feeling of dissatisfaction and meaningless cravings all the time.

To make matters worse, many of us have a strange, unhealthy relationship with food where we use it as a means to shove our stress and tensions deeper inside us so that we can enjoy instant gratification and momentary pleasure.

To live a better life, you need to change your attitudes towards food and treat it and your body with more respect. The food you eat is deserves respect, but the way you consume it only degrades it because you never realize what you eat and forget all about your meal once it is inside your tummy.

Fortunately, you can improve this by making mindfulness based eating part of your daily routine. This simple practice makes you more aware of the food you eat, how you eat it, and what it does for you. Mindful eating also trains you to do everything with an increased sense of awareness and acceptance.

How to practice mindfulness eating

Here is how you can practice it.

When it is time to have a meal, serve yourself a decent portion; it should be neither too much nor too little. If you feel like you should eat more, remind yourself that you have the option of adding more to your plate if you finish the first serving.

Sit down to eat, preferably in a quiet room and one without a TV. If possible, eat alone for a few days so as to teach your mind how to focus only on the practice and not on what is going on around you.

Say a short prayer or a few words of gratitude for your meal to appreciate and become more aware of its importance.

Inhale its aroma and focus on how that feels. Analyze it as objectively as you can and if you feel the aroma is not pleasant, accept it, but do not let that stop you from eating the meal.

Take a first, small bite, and chew it at least 20 times, and if possible, do it 32 times.

Chew it very slowly and let its flavors burst into your mouth. Focus on each flavor as you experience it and try to name it specifically. If something feels sour, think of what ingredient brings about the sourness. If you taste a sweet flavor, focus on what brought about that flavor. This simple activity immerses you more in the entire act of eating and before you realize it, you become more involved in the process and start enjoying it too.

Eat the entire meal in this manner i.e. taking small bites

and focusing on every flavor. Before taking the next bite, finish off the one in your mouth, and after every few bites, ask yourself if you need to eat more. This is important because oftentimes, we only focus on finishing whatever is in our plate and even would want a second helping or two if the meal is delicious without stopping to think if we really do need to eat that much. We have another bite ready to go even when we are still chewing the first bite.

In reality, our body does not need that much food. Unfortunately, thanks to our unhealthy and improper eating habits, we never realize this. When you stop and ask yourself if your body really needs more food and set aside your biased viewpoints, you will get a genuine answer and with time and practice (repetition), will find yourself putting the spoon down and not eating more than you need.

If you practice this meditation exercise every time you have a meal, you will find yourself eating more mindfully and with increased awareness as well as gratitude for food every time you eat.

Within a few months, your relationship with food will change and while you will still enjoy your favorite meals, you will not just eat to liv; you will start paying attention to your body while eating. Your respect for food will multiply and you will become aware of the feelings you have for food, which will ultimately help improve your eating habits as well as emotional issues such as stress and anxiety.

Chapter 9.
A Day in the Life of
a Buddhist

The teaching of Buddhism provides advice about the way Buddhists must lead their daily lives. When you wake up

You should always be in a happy and grateful state of mind as soon as you wake up in the morning. You must be grateful because you are still alive and you have a chance to face a new day. There are two main intents of any Buddhist, and these are to make the most of the day and to spend their time to improve themselves and help others. If you need to go to work, then you need to condition your mind to try and be as productive as you possibly can. Tell yourself that you must be patient and must not lose your temper. The teachings of Buddha dictate that a person must always learn to look at all the good that's around them, instead of focusing on things that cause them pain (imaginary or real). A Buddhist is always friendly to others and doesn't waste his or her time by engaging in any form of mindless chatter or gossip. Learn not to lose your patience or temper when you interact with anyone.

Morning meditation

Meditation is an essential aspect of a Buddhist's life. Usually, Buddhists tend to meditate for a little while before breakfast in the morning. The meditation session doesn't have to be a lengthy one, and it can be for five to ten minutes. The simplest way to meditate is to sit calmly and focus on your breathing. Don't concentrate on anything else other than your breath. You can use this time to gather your thoughts. You can reflect on how your life is intertwined with those of others around you. Gather your thoughts and expel any thought that isn't positive. If you feel any negative thoughts creeping up, concentrate on your breathing, and you will forget about those thoughts. Fill your mind with positivity and send this positivity to others. Try to help others. If you cannot do any good, then at least refrain from doing any damage to others.

Be mindful

Mindfulness isn't something that is merely related to meditation. In fact, if you want to live like a Buddhist, then you need to learn to be mindful throughout the day. Learn to notice any negative feelings or emotions like hate, anger, envy, greed, arrogance or anything else creeping in. Whenever you feel that the manner you act in is selfish or insensitive, then make a note of it mentally. The aim is to become aware of the situations that you are in. Most of us tend to experience self-pity at one point of time in the day or another. It is human to experience such feelings. However, you need to learn not to let any negative emotions get hold of you. Instead, you need to be mindful of what you think and the thoughts that you let into your mind. Your mind is a sacred space, and you must not fill it with all sorts of junk. When you learn to be mindful, you will learn to keep negative thinking at bay. Do you want to follow the teachings of Buddha? Well, there are a couple of things that you must keep in mind if your answer is yes. What do you do when someone criticizes you? Do you shout at them, feel bad at the rebuke or take it in your stride? Most of us tend to have a negative reaction towards criticism in any form. You need to remember that you cannot solve anything by yelling. Instead, try to calm down so that you can think clearly. You need to understand that it is a basic human tendency to desire happiness and no one wants to be unhappy. However, most people tend to be confused most of the time, and this confusion causes problems. Entertain only positive thoughts and send some positivity towards all those around you. If you think that others are open to advise, then maybe you can point out the negative aspects of their behavior. If others don't seem to be responsive, then simply stay silent. That will certainly teach you to be patient. One important thing that you must learn to control is the urge to become defensive whenever someone criticizes you. You need to remain calm and think about the criticism you receive. After a little introspection, if you feel that the criticism wasn't wrong, then you can offer your apologies and make amends immediately. If you feel that the criticism was faulty, then forget about it altogether.

Evening meditation

A Buddhist's day ends with meditation at night. You can have a short meditation session when you can recollect about all that you did during the day. To gather your thoughts, you can focus on your breathing. Use this time for self-introspection. It will enable you to think about all the good that you did and how you can improve yourself. Do you think that you lost your temper when you needn't have? Do you feel that you regret doing or not doing something? Sit down for a while and think about the events of the day. If you could, would you do anything differently? If yes, then make sure that you don't repeat the same behavior. Once you are done with meditation, the next step is to go to sleep. Make sure that you get a good night's rest before you need to tackle the next day.

You can divide Buddha's daily routine into five segments- the morning session, afternoon session, first watch, middle watch and the last watch.

The morning session starts around 4 a.m. in the morning and lasts until noon. A Buddhist's day starts at 4 a.m. and meditation follows it for an hour. After meditation, the Buddhist will try to look at the world around him and look for anyone who needs some help. The day of a Buddhist monk is simple, but it certainly isn't an easy one.

Here is an example of a day in 0the life of a Vajrayana Buddhist Practitioner.

He usually rises before six in the morning and then starts his day with meditation.

He circumambulates around his home. All over his house are shrines with statues, sacred scrolls, and other holy objects. While walking, he fingers his mala (prayer beads) while reciting a mantra.

Then, he offers 108 prostrations (bows) to show his devotion to the Buddha.

After this, the Buddhist works on whichever practice his teacher had assigned to him (e.g., visualization activity with prayer).

While he goes about his day, he chants "Om" either

silently or out loud. Meanwhile, in everything that he does, he strives to show kindness and compassion to all creatures.

In the evening, he spends a couple of hours studying the materials recommended to him by his teacher.

Then, before he goes to bed, he meditates. He also burns incense and provides other offerings at the altar.

Again, he prostrates himself before the altar and then finally, he utters a prayer for a long life dedicated to his teacher.

How to go from beginner to monk and how to master your mind

When you hear about Buddhism, what's the first thing that comes to your mind? Do you think about robed monks, incense, and huge idols? You might even believe that there is nothing in it for you, except maybe an exotic vision. However, is that what Buddhism is all about? Is there more to Buddhism than what you see in glossy magazines? Well, there is so much more to Buddhism than all that you read about in the papers and magazines. Underneath all the external trappings and trimmings, Buddhism is a way of life that can help you attain spiritual bliss.

Buddhism is usually regarded as a religion. In fact, it is a method to train the mind. It is true that it does involve monastic traditions and gives importance to ethical factors. However, it isn't limited to just that. It is not theistic because its teachings confirm that impersonal laws govern the universe and not by the hand of any creator or God. Buddha was a teacher, not a God, so there is no use for prayer, and it affirms that devotion is a means to express gratitude to its founder, and it is not an obligation. Therefore, it is safe to say that it is not a religion in the literal sense, but it is a way of life. It concentrates on methods of self-development.

A Buddhist doesn't have to have faith or even believe in anything merely because Buddha said it or because it is written in ancient texts. A Buddhist doesn't have to abide by the principles of Buddhism because it is handed down by tradition. A Buddhist can accept the Buddha-doctrine because he believes in it and because his reason finds it acceptable. It doesn't mean that everything can be rationally demonstrated, for some points lie beyond the scope of necessary intellect and require the development of higher faculties. But the fact remains that Buddhism doesn't call for blind acceptance of faith. It is a way of life that is based on the concept of training the mind. The aim of Buddhism is complete liberation from endless suffering that we subject ourselves to knowingly or unknowingly. It intends to strike at the roots of daily misery. All our acts are directed toward the attainment of happiness in one form or the other, or it is toward liberation from some dissatisfaction. Come to think of it, discontent is the starting point of all human activity, with happiness being the desired goal. If you want to learn to go from a beginner monk and learn to master your mind, then there are a couple of things that you must know.

Dissatisfaction is inescapable in en-self-ed life

The word dissatisfaction is often used to describe a lot of negative feelings like suffering, pain, sorrow and some form of displeasure. Dissatisfaction includes anything that is unsatisfactory and causes any physical suffering, mental suffering or both. One of the principles of Buddhism states that no one can escape suffering in en-self-ed life. The term "en-self-ed" life needs a little explanation. The principle essentially states that the "self" is eternal like the soul and thus has no reality per se. The core of every human being is not the soul, but it is life. Life is a constant stream of energy that changes every second. The self that we think of as eternal is, therefore, a delusion. Does this all sound confusing? The first principle is quite simple. It doesn't mean that no one can escape suffering. Instead, it means that you cannot avoid pain as long as you are stuck with the delusion of selfhood. The moment you start to think about the bigger picture, you can escape all the suffering and dissatisfaction you experience.

Craving leads to dissatisfaction

If you slip on a slippery floor and suffer an injury, you will say that the floor is the cause of your suffering. When you think about it, it does make sense to say that floor caused your pain. However, it doesn't make any sense to say that craving is the cause of your injury. The second principle of Buddhism doesn't refer to individual cases of suffering. All human beings have a self-centered craving, and this craving causes several delusions that in turn cause pain. It means that the slippery floor is an occasion for pain but not the cause. You cannot cure suffering by removing the causes of suffering. You need to try to understand the purpose of suffering and Buddhism helps with this process.

Destroy the craving

The current lives that we lead in this world are held together by all the self-centered desires that exist within us. Cravings when not satisfied cause all the pain that we experience. So, the easiest way to remove any form of dissatisfaction from your life is to eliminate all the cravings. When you destroy all delusions, you have about yourself, that's when reality comes to the forefront. One of the fundamental principles of Buddhism is to let go of all misconceptions to reveal the truth. You cannot discover reality unless and until you free yourself from any delusions you have about yourself. So, what is the reality that appears when you let go of misconceptions? The ultimate truth is the one that's full of bliss and complete freedom from all forms of suffering. According to Buddhist scriptures, the ultimate truth is the elimination of all kinds of greed, hatred, and delusion from one's mind. It is a state of being where you can finally exude complete control over your mind. Now that you know what dissatisfaction is and the causes for it, the next step is to learn to let go of this dissatisfaction that exists within us.

The way to freedom

There are eight factors that you must work on if you want to achieve independence. You need to have right understanding, right thoughts, right speech, and action in a proper manner, have the correct form of livelihood, make the right effort and incorporate mindfulness and the ability to concentrate. There is no hint of religion in any of these steps. In fact, these factors are of a psychological nature and not a religious one.

Control your mind

Dukkha means dissatisfaction, and there are different triggers that cause dukkha. It can be due to physical discomfort or even mental convolutions. The human mind is quite a complex thing, and often, all the dukkha we face starts in mind in the form of dissatisfaction caused by different triggers. The mind creates dukkha and therefore, you need to be careful about what you feed your mind. Your mind can make you happy, and it can make you unhappy too. You have the key to your happiness, and no one else can make you truly happy. All the happenings around us are triggers, and they often catch us when we are unaware. Therefore, you need to try to develop a strong sense of self-awareness. One of the simplest steps to do this is meditation. There are two forms of meditation, and they are samatha and vipassana. The former helps to make you feel calm, and the latter provides insight. If you can manage to attain some calm, then your concentration will certainly improve. If you don't use this valuable skill to gain some insight, then it is a sheer waste of time. When your mind becomes calm, you can experience joy. If your mind is calm only for a while, then the joy you experience is temporary too. The only thing that is permanent is the insight.

The stronger your sense of calm is, the more resistant it is towards all forms of disturbances. In the initial phases, even a little noise or discomfort can disrupt your calm. However, with a little practice, you can get the hang of it. Change is constant in life. You must learn to use it to obtain insight into reality. Mindfulness is an important aspect of Buddhism, and it is an integral part of meditation. Most of us tend to spend a major chunk of our lives doing different things. If you want to be able to control your mind, then you need to take some time out of your busy schedule and try to gain some insight into your mind. The mind creates our world. If your mind says you are happy, you will feel happy. It is all peachy when your mind provides you positive thoughts. However, all the trouble starts when your mind encourages negative thoughts.

If you want to achieve bliss in life, then you need to be able to control your mind. Well, the idea is to control your mind and not let it control you. When you are mindful of what you feed your mind and the kind of thoughts that it entertains, the easier it will be for you to take good care of it. Learn to treat your mind with respect and start to take care of it. Most of us tend to take our minds for granted. The mind has the capacity to do good and evil. If you want to gain a sense of control of in your life, then you need to be able to control the way your mind reacts regardless of the circumstances around you. Until you can control your mind and thoughts, you will have little control over your life. Your mind can inflict greater harm on you than any enemy of yours can. Your mind can do you more "good" than your loved ones can. Your mind can make or break your life. Therefore, it is quite important to control your mind. If you let your mind control your life, you will never be able to achieve all that you want to achieve in life. The most powerful weapon that you can wield is your mind. A mind that you can control and skillfully direct is more valuable than any other resource you possess. Meditation is just one of the means to train your mind, but not the only means. For instance, training your mind is quite similar to learning to play tennis. Initially, you will need a little help from a trainer, and then you need to keep practicing until you find your groove. If you want to learn to control your mind, then you need to put in a lot of effort and practice.

Chapter 10.
The Four Noble Truths

If you want to impress people, call it by its Pali name: Chatāri Ariya Sachānip. All Theravadans use Pali (like the way Jews use Hebrew), while Mahayanists use whatever language they're more comfortable with. This is another way to tell the different sects apart.

In The Setting in Motion of the Wheel of Dharma (the Buddha's first public discourse), the Four Noble Truths are defined as follows:

"To be born is dukkha, to grow old is dukkha, to be ill is dukkha, to die is dukkha. To come across what is unpleasant is dukkha, to be separated from what is pleasing is dukkha. Not getting the things you want is dukkha, as is the five aggregates."

It states that while there are certainly pleasant things in life, the lack of it leads to dukkha. And since birth, old age, illness, and death are an inherent part of life, then all must suffer. This is inevitable.

The Second Noble Truth explains why we suffer:

"Dukkha arises because of desire. Because of desire, we are reborn. In being reborn, we experience delight and lust. We seek pleasure here and there, we delight in sensual pleasures. We want to live, but we also want to die."

The Third Noble Truth explains how to end suffering. The Buddha taught that we have to end craving, and we have to stop developing a reliance on things. It is important to note that he did not denigrate desire.

Put simply, the Four Noble Truths can be summarized as follows:

1) The nature of dukkha: it is an inherent part of life

2) The cause of dukkha; it arises because of desire, craving, and reliance

3) To end dukkha: you have to end desire, craving, and reliance

4) How do you end desire, craving, and reliance? By following the Eightfold Path

The First Noble Truth

The Buddha did not pull his ideas entirely out of a vacuum. He was born into the Hindu religion which influenced his world views. Just as Christ was born a Jew and Jewish ideas about the nature of god and the universe therefore had a major influence on Christianity, so Buddhism is greatly influenced by Hinduism.

According to Hinduism, there is neither a heaven nor a hell. This world is it. Everything we think, say, and do affects our lives and the world around us. If they don't catch up with us in this life, they'll get us in our next birth, because Hinduism and Buddhism (as well as Jainism and Sikhism) believe in reincarnation.

Skhandha is the Sanskrit word for "pile" or "bundle," but the Buddha used it to refer to a psychological state. The Five Aggregates (Pancha Skhandhas) was therefore his explanation of why existence is dukkha.

1) Rupa (form or matter): matter is subject to heat and cold, as well as to change, decay, and damage; while form has its limitations and can therefore only do so much. As humans, we need food, drink, clothing, and shelter. Take these things away, and we cannot help but suffer. We can also be cut, burned, drowned, etc. Even if we manage to avoid these, we are subject to sickness, old age, and death.

2) Vedāna (sensation or feeling): pain is our body's way of telling us that damage has occurred, so it is only natural that we avoid the unpleasant, and desire the pleasant. The inability to control our desire for only pleasant things, however, can entrap us.

3) Saṃjña (perception or cognition): we have innate intelligence that allows us to recognize things and to discern one object, thought, or feeling apart from another.

4) Saṃskāra (personality, impulses, habits): personal experiences determine our inner, mental landscape. These result in traits that distinguish us from others. Because of saṃjña, however, we tend to prejudge things that can prevent us from trying

to understand them better, trapping us in ego and ignorance.

5) Vijñāna (consciousness or discernment): this is our innate self. Our personality changes from childhood to adulthood and old age, but vijñāna does not. This is the self that survives physical death and is carried from one incarnation to the next.

In being born, we become vulnerable, a major cause of suffering. The fact that we even long for something better, however, is due to vijñāna. It is a vestigial understanding or memory that there is something other than physical existence and its limitations.

The Second Noble Truth

Put another way, the more we want something and the more we can't get it, the more our dukkha increases. But it all begins in the mind. It is important to understand this, because herein lies the key to ending dukkha.

The terrible economy aside, even the poorest Americans generally enjoy a standard of living higher than many middle class families in the Third World. Despite this, there is a feeling of despair among many of America's poor that they are being left behind, that there is little hope for them, and so they suffer.

Surrounded by the abundance of a developed nation, and provided for by various social welfare programs, many still feel depressed. This is because they are comparing themselves to those who have far more. Even those who understand that their lives are far better off than most of the world's population, are not impressed.

For them, it is not enough to have food, drink, clothing, and shelter. They are also concerned about the quality of these things and what people might think of them. This is not to denigrate their suffering, but it does show that dukkha begins as a state of mind.

The Buddha therefore called this mental craving "taṇhā," which means "thirst." He taught that there are three types:

1) Kāma Taṇhā: kama means "desire," and while there is nothing wrong with desire, per se, dukkha arises when our thirst for pleasure and gratification becomes our sole focus.

2) Bhava Taṇhā: bhava means "internal feeling" or "mental disposition." It is the thirst for continuity: such as youth, success, personal identity, even the continuation of a relationship or state of affairs. The desire for immortality can fall under bhava taṇhā. It can also refer to a craving for wealth, power, and influence.

3) Vibhava Taṇhā: vibhava means "no becoming," "non-existence," or "extermination." At its best, it means a desire to be free from emotional pain or experiences, but at its worst, it refers to suicidal tendencies.

Since one's mental condition colors one's life, a dissatisfied mind results in a dissatisfied life. Even the rich and powerful can fall prey to vibhava, proving that it is not what one has or doesn't have that brings about dukkha. It is the mind's condition that does.

The Third Noble Truth

It is not enough to end desire, however, which is obviously impossible. The Buddha made it perfectly clear that while we are encased in flesh, we cannot help but have them. Desire is part and parcel of the human condition.

What the Third Noble Truth would have us do, though, is to investigate the causes of our desire and why we react the way we do. According to Socrates, "the unexamined life is not worth living." The language barrier aside, he'd probably get along with the Buddha.

There is a terrible misconception that a good Buddhist should go off to some monastery in the middle of nowhere and live on a single grain of rice. This is in reference to something the Buddha actually tried to do when he was starting out, and it was a disaster. It is no accident that he ended up condemning the practice of self-mortification and self-imposed hunger.

What we are asked to do is to examine ourselves, our emotions, and our reactions to things. The idea behind this is that the more we understand our motives and actions, the less we become slaves to our passions.

Why do some people turn into alcoholics, for example, but not others? Why do some people become addicted to porn while others don't? Why do some people eat and eat, knowing they're hurting themselves, but can't stop? And why do some people end up in the same deadbeat situations again and again?

These people know they're hurting themselves, but they just can't stop, even if they desperately want to. It's as if they're suffering from vibhava, and in the case of alcoholics, they probably are.

Unless we investigate ourselves, we cannot even begin to break out of our own self-destructive cycle. It gets worse. Because of reincarnation, unless we resolve our own issues in this life, we'll carry them forward into our next incarnation.

The Third Noble Truth is not asking us to turn into emotionless robots that only eat and procreate when necessary to keep us from going extinct. It is asking us to do the exact opposite.

Instead of living like zombies on automatic mode, we are being asked to look deeply into ourselves and to question our feelings and our reactions. Instead of automatically opening your refrigerator door, for example, first ask yourself: "Am I really hungry?"

Being aware of our own impulses helps us to better get a grip on them. Developing this awareness is the first step toward self mastery.

The Fourth Noble Truth

This is one of Buddhism's appeal — the promise that dukkha can end and that there are practical, doable steps to bring it about in the here and now.

The Buddha was not a god and he left strict instructions that when he died, he was not to be deified, nor were images to be made of him. To be fair, the early Buddhists obeyed this injunction, but it didn't last. According to historians, we have the Greeks to blame for this. They were the first to make images of the Buddha, patterning the classical Indian depictions of him after the Greek god, Apollo.

What makes the Buddha's message even more appealing is his insistence that we do not need to pray to gods or even believe in one; nor do we need to engage in prayers, rituals, sacrifices, build temples, or make donations to supernatural beings which need money for some reason.

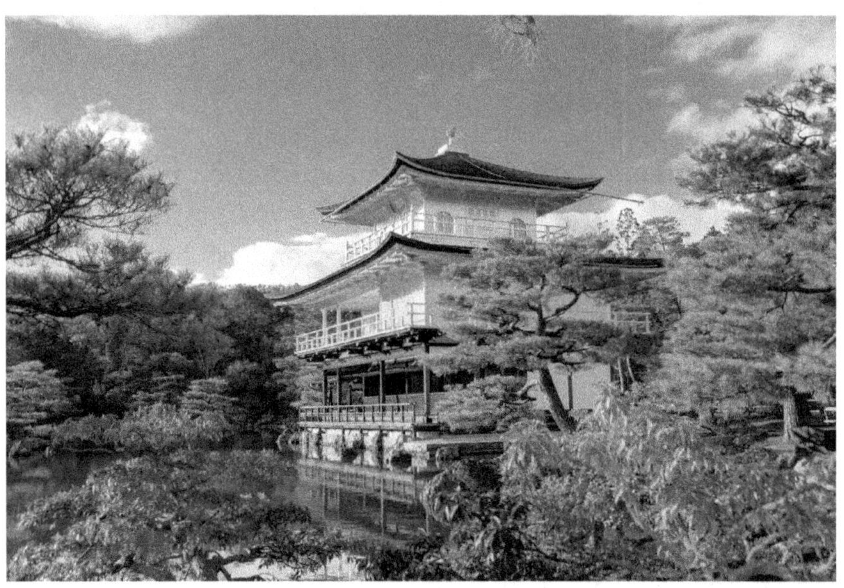

Photo: Kinkaku-ji Temple Kyoto Japan

The Buddha taught that we are all inherently powerful and that our success or failure rests on ourselves, alone:

He also made it painfully clear that he won't be there for you, nor will he ever be. He's dead, you understand?

"You yourselves must strive: the Buddhas only point the way." (Dhammapada 276)

This is the other thing that makes Buddhism different. It explains how to become Buddhas, ourselves — awakened and enlightened beings.

The Fourth Noble Truth can therefore be understood as a message in and of itself, one of hope: that there is an end to suffering, pain, grief, and loneliness.

Nibbāna, that state beyond dukkha, rests on you and you alone; not others, fate, the supernatural, or anything else.

So how do you go about it? Well, that's where the Eightfold Path comes in.

Chapter 11.
Zen Buddhism

Zen is the practice of studying your subconscious and seeing your true nature. Our true nature is devoid of past experiences and feelings or ideas that we have developed during our lives. Despite the ideas that people have about Zen being mystical and other-worldly, it is actually one of the most simple, down to earth practices around. For the most part, we are all quite ordinary on the inside. Many people believe that Zen is about having supernatural, spiritual experiences: visions, revelations, etc. In all actuality, living Zen is about experiencing regular, every day moments, with your feet on the ground, 24/7.

Zen is also the act and discipline of having undeviating experience with our lives as we are living them, day to day. It truly is the "practice of living." When we live Zen, we are fully in tune with what we are doing and have nothing unnecessary on our minds in the meantime. We are experiencing things around us just as they are.

What Zen Buddhism is NOT?

Zen is not a belief system, philosophy, or religion; it is a practice. Zen is a school of Buddhism, yet one can practice Zen without being a Buddhist. Likewise, one can be a Buddhist without practicing Zen. This holds true with all religions. We have the ability to belong to any religion we like while still practicing Zen.

Being that Zen is not belief based, therefore it is not necessary to have faith in outlandish, other worldly things that are difficult to wrap our minds around. The only thing you need to want to believe is that you have a true nature.

Zen is not about doing or attaining something. "The destination is the journey." Practicing Zen is not about reaching an end, be all goal. It is commonly thought that there is an objective to meet when studying and living Zen: enlightenment. Yet, enlightenment is not reaching some huge, mystical climax.

Zen is not about experiencing a moment of enlightenment, it is about living a lifetime of enlightenment! I will discuss enlightenment later so that you may understand it better and rid yourself of preconceived ideas tied to the word.

Zen is not about rational, active thinking. It is not about what you think. If you intellectualize anything it will hinder your practice of Zen. Instead, you need to learn how to calm and quiet your logical, thinking mind. You will be running off of intuition, which requires no deliberate effort.

Zen is not complicated, it is very simple. Zen is experiencing being alive and all that comes with it, right now. Practicing Zen may be hard for some at first, but many new things are. That is why practice is necessary. We have developed bad habits like holding on to past experiences and over-thinking everything. Bad habits take time and effort to get rid of, just like acquiring a new habits does. The process may be a little bit difficult, but not complex in the least and totally worth it.

Where Did Zen Come From?

Zen is a branch of Mahayana Buddhism. It was brought to China roughly 15 centuries ago, in 6 CE. Zen was brought to China by Indian Buddhist monk, Bodhidharma. There it was known as "Ch'an," which is the Chinese interpretation of Sankrit term, "dhyana," meaning a mind that is immersed in meditation. The term we know now, Zen, is the Japanese pronunciation of "Ch'an."

Bodhidharma went to the Shaolin Monastery in China, bringing the teachings of Zen with him. Fun fact: this is how Zen came to influence Kung Fu. Bodhidharma is still known as the "First Patriarch of Zen."

In Japan, teachings of Taoism and Buddhism were already starting to blend. Bodhidharma's lessons were along some of the same lines, so they converged easily, and were easily accepted thanks to the Tao/Buddhist influence.

Slowly but surely, many of the Indian ideas in Zen were cast off. They were slowly phased out by Chinese influences and what we commonly recognize as Zen principles. This is largely credited to Zen's sixth patriarch, Huineng. He taught at the beginning of what is known as Zen's Golden Age. The influences of this age are still taught and felt in modern day Zen, passed down in tales and the koans used for meditation.

Zen was divided into five different schools during this period. The Rinzai and Soto schools are still widely practiced today and are very distinct. I will discuss both in more detail later in this book as they are very important.

Zen spread to Vietnam early on, probably around the 7th century. Korea received Zen during the Golden Age. Because of the World War II and globalization, westerners were able to get a taste of eastern culture, including Zen. Since then, Zen has become an established practice in the West as well.

What Does Zen Teach?

Zen teachings are profoundly different from other Buddhist practices. Many Buddhists lay emphasis on the significance of researching and comprehending the historical Buddha's teachings. Contrariwise, Zen Buddhist schools stress the importance of uninterrupted, direct experience of life. We, as practitioners of Zen, are constantly trying to comprehend the significance of life. We are taught to experience life without being distracted by often unnecessary logical thinking processes, literature, or words.

Practice over Principle

In Zen, we are taught that we can only reach enlightenment and find our true nature while in a specific state of mind. We must practice putting ourselves into the proper form of consciousness. This is much more important that any written teachings or philosophies. Sure, scriptures will offer direction, but true enlightenment is found inside of yourself. In Zen, spending too much time on studying theories and principles will be a distraction, keeping our minds occupied with logical and practical tasks, actually preventing you from achieving enlightenment. Zen is also about getting rid of all the patterns of thinking and old ways of understanding in order to build new ways of seeing the reality and perceiving what really is around us and inside of us. The original Zen, as well as the genuine Buddha's intent, was free of almost any rituals, established practices, too many principles, etc. As one of the traditional folk stories says, when Buddha's students asked him what Buddhism was all about, he just raised a lotus flower and smiled in silence. They were confused and couldn't understand the simplicity and meaning behind what Buddha did. There was only one student who nodded and smiled. Buddha noticed that he understood and he passed all his simple teachings to him, and as the story goes, that's how Zen came into existence.

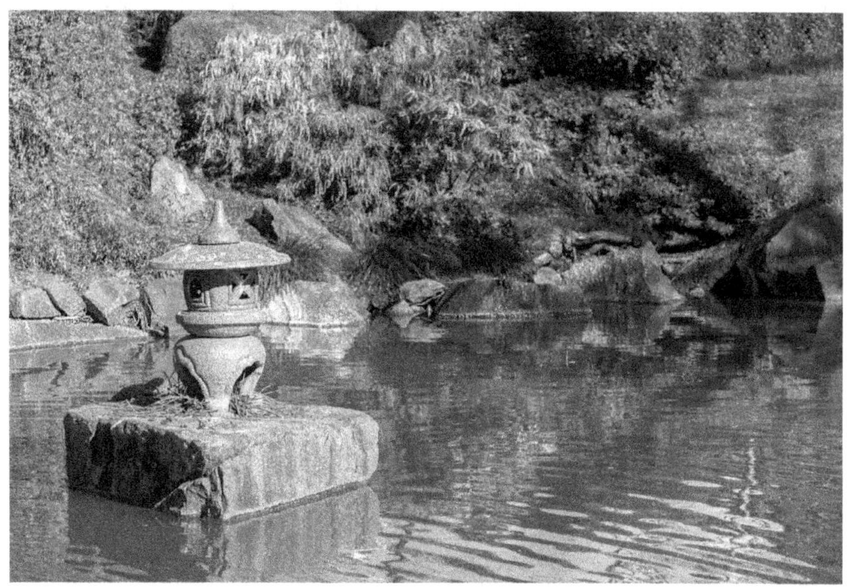

Photo: Zen garden

Meditating

Meditation is one of the most important teachings in Zen. It is key to achieving the understanding. Using Zen meditation, we put ourselves into a different state of consciousness, a higher state that allows us to live an enlightened life, not just experience a moment of enlightenment. Zen teaches you how to quiet your active, thinking mind and concentrate on becoming truly aware. While a Zen meditative state, we are conscious of our inner self and everything around us. You become an observer of your own thoughts, not actively thinking thoughts, but being aware that they are present, without necessarily judging them, repeating them or believing in them at all. Have you ever noticed how often our own thoughts are not only not real, but also not true at all?

There are two major schools of Zen Buddhism, Soto and Rinzai, both utilize different forms of mediation.

Luminous Mind

The idea of a luminous mind is a foundational teaching of Buddhism. There are a few slight variations, but the notion is generally the same. We must believe that the mind is luminous in order to gain understanding and to live an enlightened life. If we do not come to the realization that we have a luminous mind, we cannot properly train and develop them in order to function on a different level. The point being that our minds by nature are radiant, the thoughts and feelings that tarnish them are temporary. That means that we shouldn't be searching for the enlightenment and wisdom externally, as they are all already inside of us.

According to the traditional teachings of Zen Masters, the dominant feature of the new perception is to overcome all dualities: all that is either external or internal, the "me" and "not me," finiteness and infinity, being and non-being, illusion and reality, emptiness and fullness, necessity and randomness," so that "enlightened" and "not enlightened" or "liberated" and "not liberated" are the same thing. Zen teaches us that we shouldn't be looking for liberation in the "other worlds," as, in fact, this world is the "other world." That is the "satori" point of view, which is also known as the "perfect enlightenment," the "transcendental wisdom" (prajnaparamita). Does your brain hurt a little at this point? Good. Don't worry, you will ultimately understand and feel it.

We already are luminous, freed from the cycle of life and death, and already freed. Everyone already has a Buddha nature inside of them, but it is almost impossible to see and feel as our awareness is clouded and foggy. Now we just have to make our minds clear and our perception sharp enough to find this realm inside of us and connect with it.

Tarnishing thoughts and feelings will come and go. Defilements are only temporary visitors to the mind. They do not stay, nor do they permanently stain or change the mind. As long as we see it this way, believe it to be true, and analyze these things from the outside instead of actively thinking and feeling them, we can train our minds to simply observe them.

Of course, the darkness will come back, but that is why we must train our minds to let go of it. We must develop our thinking to be continuously clear. We need to acquire the ability to keep the darkness out, observe it from afar. Keeping our mind luminous is the key to ultimate happiness.

No Mind

Having no-mind, or achieving no-mindedness, is essential to living a Zen life. Too often people assume that it means to have an empty mind, when in all actuality, it is simply a state of mind that is unclouded by extensive thoughts, emotions, and feelings. When we have these things and hold onto them, we are stagnating the mind. A state of no-mind is not really still, it is constantly moving and flowing. No-mind allows us to function intuitively. It is a clean, clear, illuminating state of mind. In the Chinese understanding of Zen, we could say that it is experiencing the deepest Silence, the Primal Point of our existence - "The Road." The "No Mind" means a state that exists by itself (and which has always [forever] been there), not because of our perception, so it's not a product of our thinking and our mind.

The mind is like a mirror, reflecting the universe around us. Thoughts, feelings, and ideas are like a layer of dust coating the reflective surface of the mind. The reflection of a dirty mirror will not be clear. Yet when a mirror is dusted and clean, it shows a perfect reflection of what is in front of it. No-mind is a clean mind. This is the true state of our minds at birth. No-mind is the perfect way to function. We must clean our minds out in order to return to this perfect state.

Chapter 12.
Core principles of Zen Buddhism and simple rituals and practices that you can apply day to day

"You only lose what you cling to."

- Buddha

Achieving Zen is a very different approach to living life and is not without its obstacles or hard work. The only way to escape the negativity associated with your current self, such as greed, ignorance, and anger, is through self-realization. But, you are in luck, because Zen so happens to be the gateway through which this can be accomplished. Thesis not accomplished without effort and personal investment into the transformation, but it is possible.

Zen meditation is a crucial part of your path to enlightenment. A focus is placed on your body, mind, and breath to bring you into the present moment. When you begin, it might not be an easy task, but over time the practice will become second nature. As human beings, we are not used to taking time for ourselves. After all, there is always somebody else relying on you, right? But, if you neglect yourself, you cannot possibly take care of another person. Zen requires that you become your most important focus. You need to take the time for yourself in order to reach true happiness and understanding so you can pass those beautiful and foundational truths on to those who rely on you.

I often explain this in the same way as I explain self-love. There are people who argue against the point of self-love, but self-love isn't selfish. It's not a question of putting yourself first all the time to the detriment of others. That is selfishness. Self-love just means making yourself the best person that you can be so that you are able to give the world and the people around you the best person rather than the one who is riddled with self-doubt and who may become a liability rather than a valuable part of their lives.

Meditation is your time for yourself and should never be compromised. You are worth it, and you deserve it, whether you currently believe that or not. Setting aside the fact that meditation will be one of the main reasons for your own self-growth, meditation will help you in your everyday life. This practice will give you a tool by which to regain your calm in a heated situation. It can take only a few minutes for you to center yourself in that time and react without anger or frustration, but it takes daily practice in order to implement.

In order to practice meditation, it is important to find a clean, uncluttered area or space in which to sit. It needs to be anywhere you are comfortable and will not be disturbed by outside stimuli. It will be difficult in the beginning without having a barking dog or the neighbor's playing children disrupting your concentration, which is why outside stimuli need to be eliminated as much as possible.

Then, you need to make sure you have a comfortable place to sit. A cushion or a foam mat is usually the most popular choices, but as long as you are comfortable, then it does not matter what you use. Place your mat or cushion on the floor or a chair and make sure the air is a comfortable temperature.

Setting up an altar signifies your actualization of devotion and respect. In traditional Zen monasteries, the altar present in the meditation room is focused on the statue of Manjushri, which represents transcendent wisdom. The statue of Manjushri carries a sword, which is believed to cut away at delusions, allowing you to completely clear your mind. The image or statue you place on your home altar should be a Buddha or Bodhisattva, as it will encourage you to rid yourself of ignorance, greed, and anger. It will also help you to replace these with more positive aspirations of wisdom, peace, or compassion.

Other features that may invoke the right frame of mind for meditation are the inclusion of an incense holder and incense, a flower to evoke transient beauty, a candle to brighten your space, and water which signifies nourishment. Whatever you place or bring to your altar should be something you respect and hold in high esteem.

Meditation takes preparation as well as a change in mindset. One of the ways to focus on your mindset is to rid yourself of other physical worries. Wear comfortable, loose clothing and make sure you are rested. Tradition states that you should bow towards an altar, offer incense, and bow towards the altar again. Then, before sitting, bow towards and away from your cushion to signify your respect and intention for the practice of Zen and towards any others who may be in your presence. Then, and only then, can you take your seat.

For those with limited mobility, there is nothing against the use of a wooden chair and placing the feet flat on the floor, although the same ritual of bowing should be observed as a token of respect for the altar, the Buddha and the chair which will support you through your journey. Your hands also need to be in a similar position on your lap with your hands cupped together, palms upward and your thumbs touching one another.

While it can be hard to achieve at first, as you continue to practice you will become more flexible and find it easier to reach these positions. If neither of the above positions is feasible right now, the traditional kneeling position simply requires you to kneel with your hips resting on your ankles.

If you are utilizing a chair, that is fine. But, it is vital to maintaining a straight back. A standing position is also within reach for people who cannot sit for extended periods of time and is very simple to maintain: simply stand upright and place your feet firmly shoulder-width apart. Then, place your hands on your stomach with your right hand over your left, and lock your knees.

Whichever position you ultimately choose should be one that offers you the most comfort. You can wear loose and unrestrictive clothing since this will not distract you by causing discomfort during the process of meditation. It's vital that you understand that you need to be able to relax completely and that during meditation, you need as little distraction as is possible.

Maintaining your posture is imperative because this is the position you will hold for around 20 minutes, and correct posture ensures that you will stay comfortable and not cause bodily harm to yourself. During the meditative process, you may feel the need to move, but understand that these urges are usually a way to distance yourself from your body's energy, and this must be prevented at all costs. Recognize, acknowledge, and move through the urges. Focus on your breathing, concentrate, and you will find that these urges pass. Clear your mind, do not pass judgment on yourself, and be patient. Be sound.

Stay in this moment.

Posture plays a vital role in Zen meditation because it is imperative to find your center and relax. In order to find your center, sit forward with your hips at a higher level than your knees. Then, make sure your stomach is free to move without restriction that could potentially disable breathing. Your ears should be in line with your shoulders, and your chin should be slightly tucked in.

Then, gaze at a point just in front of you and sway from side to side in order to find your center. If you do not know what your "center" feels like, then pay attention to what is rooting you to the ground... what is keeping you from toppling over when you sway. In the sitting position on a chair, you find your center by placing your feet flat on the floor and not moving them during the meditation process. You can feel yourself become comfortable and centered.

That feeling is your center.

Breathing is the foundation of Zen meditation. Breathe normally, but with intent. As you breathe in, allow the breath to enter your body fully and pay attention to your stomach expanding. Breathe out slowly, allowing the air to escape slowly through your nostrils. You will begin to notice how the air fills your entire body from head to toe, strengthening your center and settling your mind. Count one on inhaling and two on exhaling, and continue that pattern until you have reached a ten-count.

You may find, at some point, which your mind wants to wander to other thoughts and you are no longer counting. Use this as a reminder to come back into the present moment. When you do, start again at one. After a while, you will reach a point where you can get to ten without your mind wandering, and at this point, you can begin to count to a higher number until you feel yourself wander again. Eventually what will happen is you will be able to breathe without counting at all, and your mind will never wander.

It will simply exist within the present moment.

When starting out, you may find that sitting still for twenty minutes is something you cannot achieve. Do not let this dishearten you. Even if you only manage ten minutes each day, to begin with, consistency is what matters. As your body becomes accustomed to the practice, you will find it easier to sit for a longer period and remain focused. It is important to embrace the meditation and not judge yourself. Allow the insecurities to fall away and focus on your breath, your posture, and your moment.

Each time you sit for meditation, it will be a different experience. Just like with each day you live your life, there is always something new to interpret, experience, and discover within your meditative moments. This is why it is important to keep practicing. Do not expect perfection each time. When you become distracted, take a deep breath and bring yourself back to the moment. Sometimes that requires acknowledging a thought. Why?

Because when you realize a thought, a chain can complete itself and it can fade away. In the beginning, this will almost be necessary until you learn how to teach yourself to discard unnecessary thoughts without feeling required to acknowledge them.

Then, after the meditation is complete, open your eyes and sit quietly for a few moments. Continue your breathing and allow your body to recover from the experience. Acknowledge the realizations that have come to you during your meditation and reflect on your time spent in solitude. Appreciate what you have taken from this sitting, digest the information inwardly, and then slowly rise to your feet.

If you have been standing, slowly raise your arms above your head and stretch, allowing those teachings and processed information to flow throughout your entire being.

You have now officially meditated.

Because meditation takes training and discipline, try to use every experience of meditation to further your ability, but don't consciously think of this during the meditation process. When you finish meditating, you have time to reflect on changes you can make the next time that you meditate. Let me try to give you an example.

During meditation, you felt discomfort in your legs. During meditation, we are asked to disregard this and to carry on meditating. Soon, that pain just becomes a part of the moment, and you don't notice it anymore. However, at the end of the meditation, you can make a note that next time, you try to alter the position of the cushion or wear clothing that is less restrictive. You are learning all of the time and the time that you use to make notes after your meditation is over serves as your guide for self-improvement.

Try to imagine this. You take a photograph with your camera. The settings are something you just did with your hands, but you never really took note of them. The picture that you produce is a wonderful picture, but you have no recollection of how it happened. Thus, it may be years before you learn to do that again. In the same way, meditation is an evolving thing. We know that everything is in motion in the world and that nothing is permanent. Thus, the way to increase your ability to meditate is to take a mental note of little changes that you can make to help you to get nearer to that feeling of Zen enlightenment that is the goal of people who meditate.

There are all kinds of things that can stand in the way of your meditation, but you need to know that these are all temporary as well and that today's meditation may be more successful than yesterday's or that you may have a difficult day sometimes because your mind is not yet honed to the ability to switch off external thought. That's not a problem at all and should never hinder your practice of meditation. It should still be a daily event, and when it is, you will find that it helps you enormously with so many elements of your life.

Regulating the Mind

Meditation is beneficial for physical as well as mental health. However, its primary motive is to calm your mind, declutter it and rid it of thoughts and ideas. Once your mind reaches this stage, wisdom shines like a star. Once you achieve a greater level of concentration, a state in which your mind is neither confused nor disorganized, your thoughts and negativity will start to leave you. This is why psychologists often recommend people with excessive emotional turmoil or racing minds to count their breaths before making any decisions. Counting your breath not only calms your mind, but it also calms your body and makes it more yielding. Your body becomes relaxed and free of tension, and your breathing slows down and deepens. In this stage, your mind grows calm, quiet and unperturbed.

With practice, all the impurities present in your mind start to dissolve. All the finer states in your mind vanish. Once you reach this stage, you must begin the next step-regulating mind. The last stage is to make mind ready for regulation.

There exist a variety of ways to regulate your mind, the most common being concentration. Concentrate on one single point and consider any thoughts that appear to be actors on a stage. Now leave. You will feel a sort of ecstasy in this passivity that spreads over your mind and body. Concentrate on any object you want, for instance, the tip of your nose or your belly button.

Insight Meditation

This method, though effective is still counterproductive as you are trying to counter the incrimination of ideas with another idea and thus making the whole thing redundant as you are simply replacing a negative thought with another, harmless though. Although it may sound to be a great strategy, in the world of meditation, it is futile, as you will not attain the highest level of peace unless you declutter your mind completely. You may continue to use this method as a beginner. However, you will have to forgo it when you become ready to take the next step.

We use our eyes to look at the things outside, in the next step of meditation, also known as insight meditation; you must put everything aside and try to look inside you. You must retrospect and draw your eyes towards your self and observe and find discriminating thoughts and roots. Once you find them, realize that they are worthless and you should not hold onto them. Try to dissolve or vanquish them. Once you dissolve all these thoughts, you will no longer struggle with your inner demons, and your mind will become decluttered. Developing this insight is not easy, and you need a lot of practice before you can achieve this state. Once you achieve this state, your mind disappears and is replaced by a void. This allows your mind to work flawlessly, serenely and calmly.

Beginners often report on the reduction of thoughts when they meditate, however with practice they realized that the number of their thoughts, feelings, and emotions have increased. These new thoughts are not like the old ones, as they are the feelings of realization of the 'truth' and how you can get rid of the sea of pain. Meditation can be the lighthouse that can save you from the sea of suffering and pain known as Samsara. It is as if you have suddenly lit a match in an old, dusty room and all the dirt has become visible. Thus, if you feel your mind becoming too cluttered due to meditation, don't worry, as this is the first step towards the 'Truth.' Try to abandon these thoughts while trying to preserve the insights and over time you will notice that your thoughts have started to disappear. You will be able to sense a form of profound stillness that cannot be explained in words.

Chapter 13. Conclusion Regarding Buddhism

If you were curious about Buddhism, it would pay you to watch some videos on YouTube that feature the Dalai Lama as watching the way that he behaves and the way he is disciplined is a real inspiration. For me, the Dalai Lama is a man who has discovered happiness. He is a man who spreads happiness and peace and any member of the human race can achieve that. They may never become famous or of any great significance to mankind, but that doesn't matter. The significance that they have toward others and toward themselves is what it really boils down to.

Karma is something to think about too and this means that you gain from what you reap or you get paid back for things that you do wrong. If you kill a creature, bad karma will mean that at some time, you will have bad things happen to you. If you do something that causes harm to someone else, you also have this karmic debt to pay and all men do pay this at some time in their lives. However, if you choose to live to the disciplines of Buddhism, it opens your mind to new things – helps you to feel closer to your inner self and also to the world in which you live.

Small things get put into perspective and don't grow into big things. You begin to make sense of life and want to put in the best effort that you can. Even for people with strict religious beliefs, Buddhism allows development of understanding and will make you a better Christian, a better Hindu, a better atheist or a better person because the disciplines are all about living your life to the full, without suffering unhappiness and distress. When you are able to do that, the joy that you spread to the world around you and the respect you give to yourself are one and the same. That's when you know you have found something of deep value – something that Siddhartha Gautama found 2500 years ago and wanted to share with the human race.

For those who have read this book with an "open mind" to learn as I have requested in the introduction, I congratulate you. By now I believe you will realize that this book goes in-depth on the essential teachings of Buddhism and how one's life can be improved through them.

Think back to your thoughts and perceptions about Buddhism before you read this book. I hope this book has been able to answer some question and help you know more about what Buddhism is all about. If you still have other questions that have not been addressed thus far, you can read further in the references provided at the end of this book.

Lastly, I wish you success as you try out a few take-home lessons from this book to enhance your lifestyle.

However, you need to be consistent with whatever you want to attempt. I hope you become a better person in all facets of life based on the teachings you have learned from this book. I look forward to reading testimonials about how this book has impacted your life positively. I am itching to read your success story. Cheers!

Chapter 14. Introduction to Yoga

I'm sure that a lot of you think that since yoga is an old set of beliefs that not only was it first conceived in India, but the history of yoga also must feature significant events where many of the initial founders of yoga came into contact with other Asian inhabitants from territories outside the borders of India. This conviction might also lead some of you to reach the conclusion that perhaps yoga borrowed and, in some cases,, integrated ideas as a direct result of the Indian founders of yoga interacting with spiritual individuals who hailed from other parts of the Eastern hemisphere. Of course, it's understandable that many of you would harbor such thoughts about yoga, especially those who have never even taken a class centered on the teachings of yoga or when conversing with someone you chose to conceptualize your own interpretation of what yoga resembles in your own mind.

For many people, the very idea of starting yoga stems from such imagery because it is these vivid images that are perhaps incredibly enticing to many who wish to give yoga a try while for others, the word yoga is connected to the idea of being a challenge that would aim to push him or her outside the bounds of their own comfort zone.

True, the history of yoga might not resemble the kind of history that is linked to the progression of a country such as the United States over a prolonged period of time that measures how various circumstances and factors compelled the country to shift its gears while continuing to develop its identity as a nation as a whole, but that does not mean that the history of yoga should be seen as something that you can just brush off. There are many details that are worth examining because each of the factors that have occurred in the past has determined the present-day fascination and even the obsession with what yoga has to offer. Thus, it is extremely imperative to examine yoga from a much deeper level in terms of analyzing its historical background as this is the best way that a person can develop a much more enriched and nuanced comprehension on how yoga has been able to spread all over the world and become something that many people native to American soil love to partake in.

There is a lot of mystery concerning the origins of yoga because when yoga was first implemented the writings that were correlated to yoga were conducted on palm leaves that were not exactly the sturdiest of materials to write on, thus a lot of what was written was susceptible to inevitable destruction, either in the form of disappearing, undergoing severe vandalism, or being consequently obliterated. Though there have been roughly 5,000 years of progress with regards to yoga, some people who have conducted studies on this have found that yoga is perhaps even older, stretching back as far as roughly 10,000 years into the past. Due to this fact, it is important that yoga's history is separated into several major periods of time, which are connected to its birth, progress, and the people who would begin to follow its prominent teachings. While it is obvious that it began several years ago, around 5,000-10,0000 years to be more precise, the location in which yoga was conceived is also important to keep in mind.

The era in which yoga first emerged is known as the pre-classical period, and while it is true that yoga was developed on the Indian subcontinent, the region in which yoga was first cultivated was within the northern part of India; however, it should be noted that it was founded by a specific ancient civilization that is known as the Indus-Sarasvati. Despite the point mentioned earlier about how yoga was imprinted into the less sturdy material of palm leaves which has contributed to shrouding much of yoga in mystery, yoga has been mentioned in stronger material as well, such as a collection of written work that is considered to be quite old and is known as the Rig Veda. What is the Rig Veda?

Chapter 15.
History of Yoga

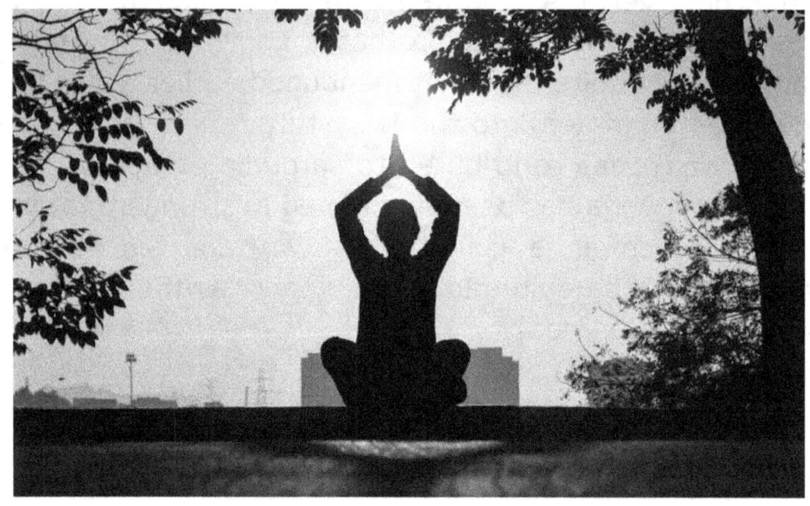

Yoga is incredibly and increasingly popular. This is because yoga is amazing. When most Americans hear the word "yoga" they think of the stretches and postures called asana (āsana) that come to us from Hatha Yoga, and a well-rounded asana practice is indeed uniquely healing. In fact, it saved my life, which you can read all about in my first book, Yoga to Ease Anxiety.

There is, undeniably, an emphasis on the physical in American yoga culture. Even when the philosophy is taught, it's usually from the perspective of how we can apply it to our lives today. This approach is super useful, but the teachings themselves are often taken out of context, which can lead to some confusion. What I hope to offer with this book is an introduction to the story of yoga, its history, and its philosophy in a linear way that is accessible to contemporary teachers and students of yoga.

It is not my intention to tell anyone what they have to believe or what they should or should not do in order to be a yogi or yogini (yoginī). I just want to relate the history of yoga and yogic ideas in a casual, relevant way.

It's taken me a long time to feel like I know enough to share this information. I first became interested in Eastern philosophies as a teenager after reading the Transcendentalists and Beat poets. As an undergrad, I was a Religious Studies major in a department that took a historical approach, and as a grad student I studied mysticism.

When I decided I was going to commit to the practice of yoga, I read everything about it I could find. And when I decided to do a 200-hour teacher training, I simultaneously enrolled in an 800-hour course in the History, Philosophy, and Literature of Yoga with the great yogic scholar Georg Feuerstein. I felt that if I were going to represent the tradition, I'd better understand it.

When yoga began, it was taught from one teacher to one student, both of whom had renounced the world in pursuit of spiritual liberation. I've been fascinated by the question of how yoga went from that intimate and dedicated scenario to hour-long classes at the local Y. As a teacher, I have continued to bump up against questions, situations in modern yoga that make no sense when compared to its austere history. So, I kept reading, researching, and trying to find answers. I've also spent the last few years serving as faculty for teacher trainings, where students often come up with some of the toughest and most interesting questions. Now I believe I have enough of the puzzle together to share it with others.

It's important to me to present an accurate picture of the yoga tradition. It's also important to me to present the information in a way that is relatable. That's how it goes with yoga: its history is so vast and compelling that when you walk through one door you enter another room full of doors. I make no claim to being comprehensive; that would be impossible.

I also make no claim to objectivity. This is the product of my investigation into the spiritual path I practice and teach. I weave the history of asana throughout the book because it's of interest to American yoga. And the texts I examine are the ones American yoga culture deems important. The translations I use are those that are accessible, as in both easily acquired and easily understood, or at least easier to understand than some of the more academically oriented translations.

My intentions and hopes are to provide a general history, to relate the fundamental philosophies of the yoga tradition, to tell the story of how yoga became what it is and made its way to America, and to spark interest and further investigation into this awesome, kaleidoscopic subject.

Our Map

The history of yoga gets wily in spots. In the beginning there are long stretches of homogeneity and then there are flurries of new ideas and cultural experiments. In the last three hundred years, yoga has been shaped in part by cross-cultural influences and interconnections. And more recently, dozens of individual personalities have grafted their own particular styles onto the tree of yoga.

To better organize our journey, we'll need a map. What follows is one of several possible approaches to categorizing the main events in the history of yoga. I find it to be the one that makes the story the most intelligible.

Upanishadic Age (1500 – 1000 BCE). The Upanishads are early texts that provide the ideological roots of yoga.

Epic Age (1000 – 100 BCE): In "Great Warriors and the Age of Epics," we'll enter the stories of larger-than-life heroes and avatars. We'll examine the two illustrious epics of India, the Ramayana and the Mahabharata, for their contributions to yoga.

Because this is a book about the history of yoga, we will pay a lot more attention to the past than to the present. While we'll take a minute at the end to look at the issues and potential of modern-day American yoga, only time will give us the perspective to tell what trends will have a lasting influence.

Throughout the book, we will be covering more horizontal ground than vertical. That is to say, we won't be diving very deep into any one subject. Again, my intention is to provide an overview, an understanding of the big picture of yoga, and hopefully pique your interest in delving further into one area or another.

Along the way, we just might find that there is both a lot more and a lot less that historically falls under the umbrella of yoga than what is represented as doing so today. To show respect for the tradition and to avoid cultural misappropriation means first knowing what is and is not original to it.

Furthermore, for practitioners, having a clear understanding of yoga's history helps us to see our own experiences in context. As Feuerstein put it, "To learn about the historical evolution of Yoga is more than an academic exercise; it actually furthers our self-understanding and hence our efforts to swim free of the boundaries of the ego-personality."

A Word about Words

Yoga comes to us from Sanskrit, which is the sacred language of the Hindu tradition. Sanskrit is an ancient language that derives from the same Indo-European family of languages as English, which is why we come across cognates every once in a while. "Yoga" is one of them. It means the same as the English word "yoke."

There's a lot of Sanskrit in this book. The first time we see a new Sanskrit word (and sometimes the second if they are far apart from one another) it will be italicized. And the first time we see a word that's in the glossary it will be in bold. There are a lot of words that are both.

At the moment, there are a few different standards for expressing Sanskrit words in English. One is to use the International Alphabet of Sanskrit Transliteration (IAST), which has lots of diacritical marks—lines and dots and tildes—on letters to signify how a letter should sound and which syllables should be emphasized. IAST is informative if you know what you're looking at, but not everybody does.

Another option is to give it our best go using just the plain old Roman alphabet. My compromise between ease of reading and wanting to be as accurate as possible is to list them both, if they are different, on the first usage of the word. I've put the IAST version in parentheses, as I've already done with (āsana) and (yoginī) above. After that, I use just the naked letters.

I would absolutely recommend spending some time with an online pronunciation guide with audio to learn how the words are supposed to sound. I like the one yoga teacher Tilak Pyle provides,[5] but you may find something that suits you better.

Chapter 16.
What is Yoga?

I bet if you walked into your workplace right now, and asked how many people practice yoga, about one-third of your workplace would raise their hands. Yoga is incredibly popular today and there are many people who practice it. From your grandmother to your dog walker, there are at least two people in your life who practice yoga. If you're reading this book, it's likely that you practice yoga, or you're interested in practicing it. You're not alone. There are roughly 36 million people in the U.S. who practice yoga, and that's a statistic from three years ago (Wei, 2016). Could you imagine how many people practice now? The answer is a lot. I know that's not scientific, but it's a lot. You can't even drive around a city block without seeing a yoga studio.

Yoga is a practice that is enjoyed across the lifespan. Children, teens, adults, and seniors can all enjoy the benefits of yoga and there are classes and practices dedicated to each age group. While we generally see young, thin women in yoga ads, yoga is enjoyed by everyone. In fact, middle-aged adults and seniors practice yoga far more than youths. If you are healthy and fit, or not, you can still benefit from yoga practice.

Despite all the popularity and the endorsements from

celebrities about the wonder of yoga, it's hard to know exactly what yoga is exactly. After all, is yoga just stretching? How is it different from other stretches? What makes it so popular?

Yoga is a detailed, beautifully historic practice. When I say, 'meditative exercise,' I use the phrase to show both aspects of yoga. Yoga can be used for mindfulness and meditation, but it's also used for physical exercise. So, there are often two parts to yoga, the physical and the spiritual. Let's look at both parts.

Most of us are aware of yoga as an exercise. When you go to a mainstream yoga class, this is what you typically get. Yoga for exercise is all about moving your muscles and holding stretches to increase your flexibility. It doesn't really matter what type of yoga you do, there is always this element of stretching and some holding, even if it's only for a breath. Whether your practice is slow or fast, you'll have poses that align your body in certain ways to give you relief, or to cause you to stretch tight muscle groups. By the end of many yoga sessions, you feel loose, light, and often relaxed. If you're doing an active practice, you may even feel worn out.

Yoga works with all muscle groups. For beginners, most of your poses are going to focus on the legs, arms, hips, and some chest poses. Once you move to more advanced poses, you start to work on all parts of your body, stretching your back, shoulders, abdominals, and more. You can even do yoga that focuses on your hands, feet, neck, and head. So, yoga can activate as many muscles as other kinds of physical exercise.

There is a strength component to yoga, though it's more subtle than say lifting weights. This is because it uses your own body weight to increase your strength. People can often add extra parts to yoga for increased strength development, but for the most part, your body weight in specific poses is all there is. The poses help your body to build more strength in each muscle group. They also help to increase your flexibility by reducing muscle stiffness. Of course, just like many other exercises, depending on the type of yoga you do, you may walk away from the session and be sore the next day.

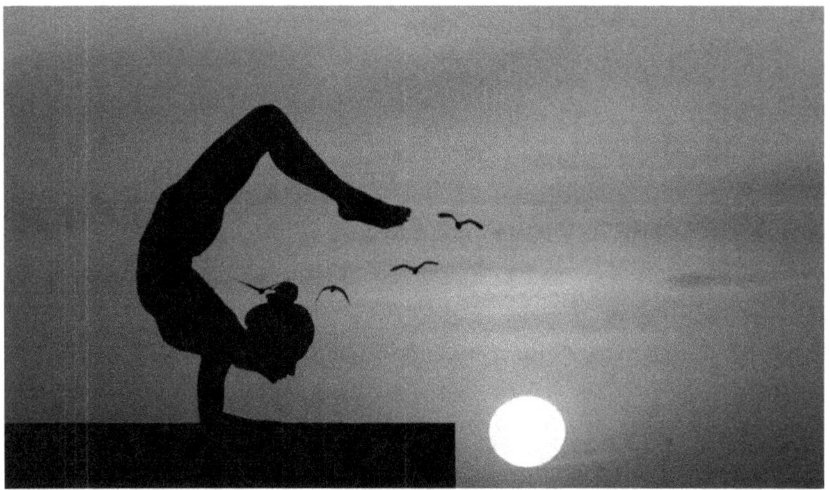

While most of us see yoga as a strength building or flexibility building exercise, it's also a cardio-vascular exercise. Cardio exercises, often called aerobics, help improve your heart health and circulatory health. Running, cycling, and swimming are all exercises that get your heart racing and in turn help to improve your cardiovascular health. Yoga can also do the same. While there are many slow yoga practices, there are also some very intense ones. There are yoga practices that move very quickly, moving from pose to pose and putting you in strenuous positions. These often cause your heart to race and for you to start sweating as you strain in each position. This cardiovascular benefit is even better if the practice is done for a long duration (think an hour-long class instead of a 15 minute one). So, yoga can also be considered a cardiovascular exercise if it's done with that goal in mind.

The breath also plays a key role in the physical aspects of yoga. You'll often find when you do exercise that you breath as you like. More often than not, you're breathing shallowly and rapidly if you're doing cardio and sometimes you might even hold your breath when you do other kinds of exercise. In yoga, there is emphasis on the breath, your aim could be to breathe slowly, or sometimes quickly, but always deeply. This helps you to maintain focus as you go through your poses, but also helps connect each movement to a breath. This means that your timing is naturally orientated. It also helps you to truly focus on the 'hows' of your practice. You start to pay more attention to the movement of your shoulders or hips, how your back is positioned, or the angle of your joints. All of this can lead to better, safer, pose positions, but also help strengthen the rest of your body.

So, yoga is a physical exercise that goes beyond just stretching. It offers strength and flexibility training and cardiovascular training. These things are more than just average stretching which most newcomers expect. Incorporating the right breathing also brings you better stability and balance, which are important to most exercises.

Beyond the physical aspects of yoga are the mental and

spiritual aspects. Mentally, yoga practice can put you in a 'zone'. You know the zone I'm talking about. It's the zone of perfect focus. Maybe you've experienced the 'zone' at work, when you're working on a perfect project and you are utterly focused on your task. This focus helps you to achieve more. In different circumstances, it can help you engage with others and to quiet the anxiety in your mind. This focus is incredibly beneficial. During a yoga practice, you might find yourself slipping into that perfect 'zone', where your mind is quiet, and you are fully focused on your body's movement. A lot of people call it a sense of peace when they practice, whether it's a slow yoga practice or a quick one.

Yoga also provides another aspect to that focus. It often provides awareness. Awareness is not just a general awareness of the events in the current day. In combination with focus, awareness means that you are aware of your present moment, what is happening around you and inside of you. This presents a type of clarity. Instead of thinking about what you are going to do later in the day, or stressing about what you did the day before, you are placed in this present moment. A consistent yoga practice can often lead to this moment. So, yoga can increase your focus and awareness inside practice, but these are lessons you can also carry with you.

A key part of achieving awareness and focus during yoga practice is your breathing. By actively choosing to focus on your breathing, you move the function from one that's automatic to one that is consciously thought about. This is very similar to mindfulness, where you focus on the breathing and exclude some of the other thoughts in your mind. Yoga can put you into a mindful state while you are practicing. By focusing on the breath and poses, you move your mind away from emotional stress and focus it instead on the present moment and actions. This results in that feeling of being 'lifted' that many people feel after doing a yoga session. That being said, you don't want to focus on the breath so much that you end up feeling drained at the end of the session. Balance is key.

The mindfulness and meditative aspects of yoga are closely related to spirituality. Spirituality is different from religion, though they do tend to be mistaken for one another. Spirituality is about your connection to the fundamental life questions. Mindfulness and meditation can be a part of spirituality. They can also be a part of religion if you practice a religion where mindfulness and meditation are encouraged. Religions, unlike general spirituality, is about your connection to a fundamental power and usually includes religious texts and rituals. If you are religious, it generally (though not always) affects your spirituality. But if you're spiritual, that doesn't necessarily mean you're religious.

I don't really want to get into the philosophical aspects of religion and spirituality. Suffice it to say that activities that help clear the mind, like yoga, are often considered to be a part of spirituality since they take you beyond yourself and instead help you focus on the moment now. Yoga is only spiritual if that's how you want it to be. For many people, they only want the physical aspects of yoga, and others practice purely for the spiritual or religious aspects.

Whatever your reasoning for practicing yoga, you can call it an exercise that is both physical and spiritual, which moves it a bit beyond your typical exercise experience.

Chapter 17.
The Eight Limbs Of Yoga

Yoga Sutras of Patanjali, an old and solid wellspring of Yoga, alludes to eight limbs of Yoga or Astanga in the Sanskrit dialect. Every last limb is a successive step towards a healthier and even more satisfying life; and asana is only one of these back to back steps. Alternate limbs are the accompanying:

- Yama - this one comprises of rules identified with good conduct towards the group.

- Niyama - this one as well, comprises of rules identified with good conduct towards you as a person.

- Asana - simply like we have as of now seen, Asana is the practice of physical stances and postures.

- Pranayama - this one includes the rehearsing of solid breathing activities.

- Pratyahara - this one includes the withdrawal of all faculties and disposing of any diversions from the outside world.

- Dharana - this one includes focusing and concentrating on something without getting occupied by anything, be it outer or inner.

- Dhyana - this one includes reflection.

- Samadhi - this one expands upon Dharana and it concentrates on the converging of the individual and the universe.

Yoga Is Not a Religion

The vast majority partner yoga with religion, yet in all actuality Yoga is NOT a religion.

This is on the grounds that it doesn't direct or propose a divine being to be worshiped. Religion can be depicted as an association or affiliation where they adore a divinity or gods through conventional ceremonies. This incorporates examining antiquated writings that include an ethical code, which they withstand to under the direction and authority of an appointed person.

The individuals who have practiced Yoga can say that Yoga does to be sure have something in the same manner as religion; for instance, there is the investigation of old writings and the get-togethers to examine under an accomplished pioneer. Notwithstanding this, these two alone, don't make up a religion; regardless of the way that there are some Yoga practices that do advance intercession on an all-inclusive soul, which is at times alluded to as god.

Yoga assigns conventional physical and mental orders

beginning in India. Hot yoga is the same teach yet practiced in climes that are no less than 105 degrees Fahrenheit. Bikram's yoga is practiced in hot situations also yet there are particular arrangements of movement's poses numbering 26 aggregate. It centers upon the development of a sound personality and body, and on accomplishing mindfulness. The different practices and controls of yoga are accessible to everybody, regardless of what their way of life or conviction frameworks. Yoga practice likewise includes creating all inclusive mindfulness and individual refinement through the yamas and niyamas, a progression of morals and controls proposed to develop living in amicability with others and in unity with our actual selves.

Yama - Yamas are moral teaches that identify with how we ought to live in a mutual world with peace and respectability. Niyama - These controls identify with the individual and concentrate on living a solid, satisfied and mind-blowing life. Asana - The word asana implies to be', in the feeling of being in a stance. The asanas were produced for the support of a sound personality and body, with every stance influencing the body, brain and feelings in a one of a kind ways and filling in as a pathway to adjust and wellbeing. Pranayama - In the practice of pranayama, we create breathing systems that build oxygen allow and reinforce lung limit while likewise expanding the retention of prana, or life force. In its most straightforward form, pranayama includes profound, full relaxing. With consistent yoga practice of yoga, you will get quality, adaptability and great wellbeing, the advantages of which stream into all parts of life. Expanded vitality levels bring another point of view on life, the incrassated emotions of self-esteem and motivation lead us to find abilities and intrigues we never knew existed and issues that once appeared to be overpowering turn out to be more reasonable.

Yoga is an old profound way. At its embodiment it implies union. There are a wide range of perspectives or limbs inside of the way of yoga. Asana, or the physical part of yoga has increased expanding notoriety in the North America. Most understudies who practice yoga to do as such at yoga studios, yet regularly enthusiasts fancy a space to practice their yoga at home. On the off chance that you are considering setting up a space for yoga, you don't have to do any significant upgrades that will impact the structure or re-deal estimation of your home. Keep with the straightforward embodiment of yoga and you will make a room that suits your needs and won't oblige real remodels.

Quite a bit of yogic logic is considering adjust, straightforwardness and simplicity of effort. Consider these qualities when drawing closer your new yoga room and its style.

Pick a room in your home that has enough security. A room with an entryway that closes is ideal, so you can enter your space and have relative protection amid your practice. Likewise, consider a room that has a sufficient measure of characteristic light. The biggest redesign, you may need to consider is the establishment of hardwood or stopper floors. Effectively covered floors are additionally adequate.

Preferably, you need to pick a room that gives you enough space to extend on the floor longwise. The roof ought to be sufficiently high to permit you to remain on the tips of your toes with your arms extended as high overhead as you can reach. In the event that there are certain to be a greater number of yogis than yourself in your room, consider that these estimations should be duplicated by the quantity of members.

You will require a wardrobe or a racking unit for capacity of yoga props, for example, mats, reinforces pieces, straps and eye packs. Here, you may need to store yoga writing and maybe a sound framework, if you appreciate honing to music or utilizing guided practice discs.

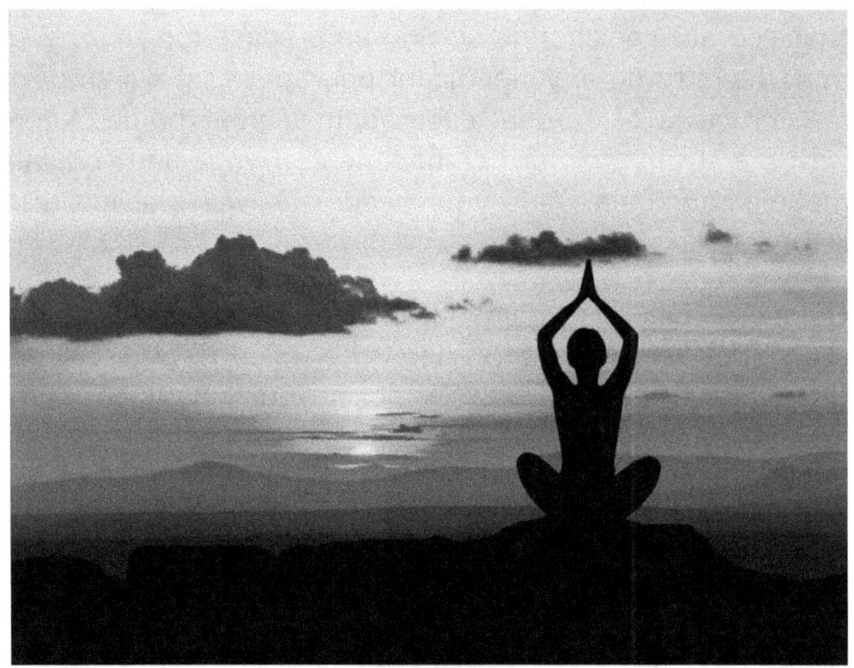

At the point when painting your yoga room considers shading that inspires quiet. Look to nature to move you shading sense of taste. A decent place to begin is with hues in the delicate green and blue hues. You can then embellish the dividers with sprinkles of shading maybe a most loved yoga notice, a cutting or possibly some request to God banners close to a window. If you do a livelier form of yoga, you may need to look to a more outlandish and energizing sense of taste of reds and purples to move your practice. Imagine a room that reflects you and your practice and that in a perfect world stays consistent with the stylistic theme of your whole home.

Make central focuses. Spot candles, statues, cards and photographs in places that are significant to you in your practice. Scan for pieces that inspire an inclination of center and cool. At all times, maintain a strategic distance from any jumble in your room.

Chapter 18.
What Yoga Can Bring
in Your Life?

The joints are a location, a joining, they are the place in which two bones connect. These joints can be immovable, such as where the bones of your skull connect or like where the six bones that make up your pelvis meet together. However, more frequently we categorize joints as slightly or fully movable. This includes joints such as many joints within the spine, the three in the wrist, or even the larger single joints like your hips, knees, elbows, and shoulders.

First, we need to look at the anatomy of a joint. Just because a joint is two bones connecting doesn't mean there isn't anything else making up your joints. Your joints are not merely two bones poking and prodding each other. Instead, they have components to help connect them, so that your body can work as a fully mobile unit.

Along with the bones, your joints are also made up of tendons connecting the muscle to bone, ligaments to connect the bones together, cartilage to help cushion the bones and prevent them from grinding up on each other, and synovial fluid. The purpose of this fluid is to act as lubrication so that your joints don't create friction, get stuck, or cause damage to any of the components.

When a joint is healthy all of its components work in harmony with a full range of movement. This results in a perfect slide between the adjoining bones in which the pressure is evenly distributed to prevent injury. Usually, there won't be pain, as there isn't excess cartilage fragments and it has the proper amount of synovial fluid.

On the other hand, if a joint is unhealthy is really frequently result in pain. What causes a joint to be unhealthy? If any single component of the joint is not properly working, it is a problem. This means if there is too little synovial fluid, if there are excessive cartilage fragments, if a ligament or tendon develops a tear, or if the bones themselves are damaged.

One of the most common causes of joint damage is osteoarthritis. This is a degenerative disease of the joint where the cartilage in the joints begins to wear and break down, causing the bones to grind together with friction. The result is pain, inflammation, and a loss of motion.

Contracture.

Even people without osteoarthritis experience damage and pain in their joints. One common example of this is when people experience contracture, which is when the joint loses mobility, it is a shrink wrapping of the joints. There are many potential causes of this condition, such as illness, cartilage or ligament damage, muscle atrophy, and nerve damage. One of the most common causes of contracture is a problem in the ligaments of your joints.

As we go about life, we can develop tiny microscopic

tears in your ligaments. These tears are so small that they aren't even visible on the strongest of magnetic imaging scans. All the while, these microscopic tears still cause small wounds that must be healed by adding in new ligament tissue where it is missing, in much the same way that you might add in a missing piece on a puzzle.

It has long been known that your ligaments function by healing in this way. But, it for a long time it was a mystery why your ligaments don't end up too long if they form tears, fill with more ligament tissue, and repeat. After all, if you stretched a piece of saltwater taffy and every time it tore added in more taffy you would have an ever-growing taffy piece. The taffy would simply get longer and longer as it would never stop stretching, tearing, and patching.

In search of an answer to this ever-puzzling question, Professor Laurence Dahners of the University of North Carolina found the answer. What he found resulted in a groundbreaking discovery. In turns out that the body has a function which works as shrink-wrap, which coats your joints and works on removing any extra ligament material so that they don't become too long. There is one part that maintains and creates the material for your ligaments and another part that actively removes excessive material. We see this pattern all over the body, there is a similar aspect that works in your bones in which osteoblasts work to create bone tissue while osteoclasts dissolve bone tissue. It is a give and take, once again Yin and Yang.

You can actively witness the examples of this shrink-wrapping ligaments in your own life. Think back on a time when you were injured, maybe you sprained your arm or broke your foot. You were likely put in either a cast or a sling for a number of weeks or months. When it comes to time to take the sling or cast off you find that your arm or leg don't move as easily as it once did. Now, your joint is moving more slowly, and it feels stiff; it might even "freeze" in place stuck for a moment. This is because as you were not stretching and using your ligaments the body naturally took away what it saw as excess material that you weren't using. When it was time to once again resume normal use of your limb you felt the lacking ligament. Thankfully, this is never a problem. Sure, your limb may be stiff for a day or two, but, as you go about usual use of your limb the ligament will stretch and any microscopic tears that form in the process will be filled in until your ligament is back to its usual length.

Of course, some people experience contracture without first developing an injury and having their joints immobilized for a period of weeks. This can happen when you naturally limit your own mobility. For instance, if a person who has practiced yoga daily for years and someone who has never attempted yoga both attempted the same yoga pose or asana, then obviously the person who had never practiced yoga will be much stiffer and less flexible. That person simply will not have the same range as the experienced yoga student.

The good news is that you can easily and naturally treat contracture all by practicing Yin style yoga. While the muscles get their best workout from rapid movements, such as cardio, ligaments get their best workout from still stretching, by applying a traction, which as you know is one of the basic definitions of Yin yoga. In fact, if a person stretches too quickly, as can happen in Yang yoga, it can cause the ligaments to tear too much, resulting in injury, inflammation, and pain.

Because you stretch your ligaments too much, if you quickly move it will disrupt them while they are in a vulnerable state, causing injury. This is why we always stress the importance of slow movements not only entering the pose but exiting the pose, as well.

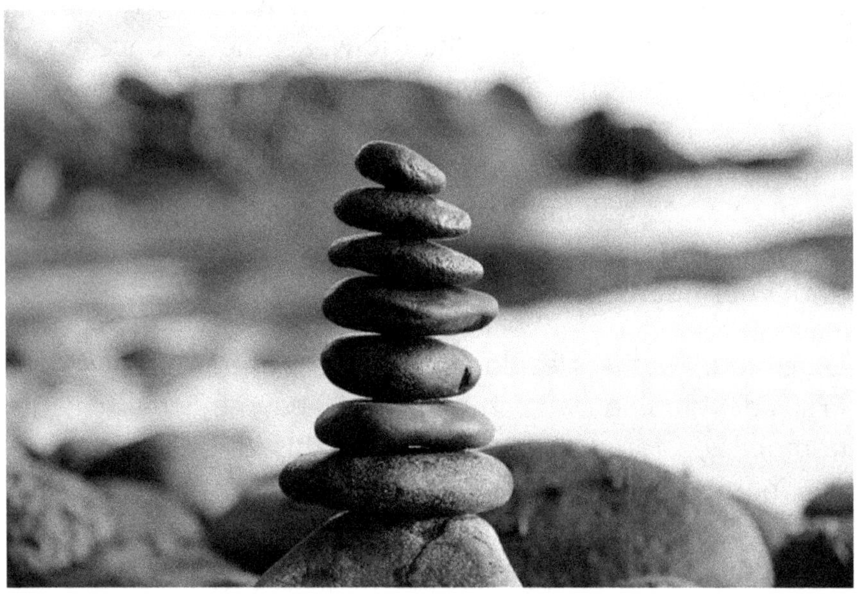

Fixation.

We all hear a snap, crackle, and pop come from your bodies occasionally when we move. While most people know that these can be caused by friction and the release of gas, many people are unaware of the third cause: fixation.

Sometimes, there will be a bubble of nitrogen that forms in this synovial fluid. When these bubbles release you hear a pop, this is the release of gas that causes popping. Whenever this happens, it will be a while until you can pop the joint again, as there are no more bubbles in it.

Friction happens when two surfaces of the joint rub against each other, and it can happen repeatedly in a row without a break in-between. Just as you may press your finger and thumb together to snap, therefore making a sound with friction, a similar reaction can happen within your joint. This happens when tendons, ligaments, or cartilage temporarily becomes stuck, causing it to press together until it can no longer hold and then firmly releasing with friction, causing the same snapping sound within the joint. A good example of this is when a person cracker their own knuckles or a doctor cracks someone's neck.

The final cause, and greatly unknown by many people, is fixation. But what is fixation? Put simply, it is when two surfaces temporarily become fixed together, it is the temporary joining together of two surfaces. When the two surfaces become unstuck and release, the resulting sound or popping is the creaks and pops we all hear in your own joints from time to time. Often, the pops you experience when you go into a yoga pose is a result of this fixation. Usually, the resulting pop causes a feel-good pressure release.

There are three conditions that must be met in order for fixation to take place:

First, both surfaces must be smooth. This means that your bones are the perfect material to become fixed to each other, as they are smooth. It wouldn't work if they were textured like sandpaper.

Second, there must be a fluid acting as a lubricant between the two surfaces, just as it happens in our joints.

Thirdly, the two surfaces must be under enough pressure

to push them together.

Many of us experience fixation in a variety of ways in your everyday lives, and not just within your bodies. For instance, if you are washing dishes you might find that two pieces of silicone become fixed together. This happens because the silicone is a smooth surface, there is water to act as a lubricant, and as you are handling the material you apply the pressure. The two pieces of silicone then become temporarily fixed and must be separated. The same principle carries out in your joints.

There are very good reasons for caring to break this fixation. Firstly, it feels good as it releases the pressure between the two bones. But, more importantly, it is not healthy for the bones to maintain fixation for long-term periods. If bones become fixed within the joint and we do not remove the fixation, then the two bones can become fused together. The result would be an immovable joint, that would require surgery to gain use of again. Thankfully, we can prevent this from ever happening by releasing the fixations naturally and easily. When you practice Yin yoga you are moving the joints just further than you usually would, which applies just a bit of pressure to the joint, allowing the fixation to dissipate and the pressure to release.

Chapter 19.
Practice

Yin yoga is based upon the Hindu teachings which endorse the idea of a triumvirate of Gods. These three gods, Brahma, Vishnu and Shiva are responsible for building, preserving and destroying the world. This process is seen as a necessity to ensure that change is always present, and the world becomes a better place. As such Shiva, the destroyers are seen as both Yin and Yang, a good force and a bad force.

This teaching may seem a little mystical in nature, particularly in comparison with the modern world and the amount of scientific research illustrating the existence or non-existence of gods. However, the principle behind this story is what matters and what is still true today.

As you start to explore Yin yoga and use it to look inward, at your own beliefs, fears and desires you will realize that the negative things which you hold onto need to be released and are actually good things, not bad. Destruction and negative issues are essential to generating a healing environment; confronting these issues will allow you to learn and flourish as an individual. This is one of the core principles of Yin yoga; the ability to know yourself and listen to both your own mind and the world around you. Indeed, through the pain of destruction comes the beauty of healing and new beginnings.

Yin yoga can provide you with the strength to carry on through difficult times and allows you to work through the emotions that come with difficult situations, emerging the other side as a stronger, more balanced person.

The passive exercises which are now known as Yin yoga are a part of ancient Chinese and Indian history. It was originally used to still the mind, allowing meditation and focus for other parts of a training program. These exercises still work in the same way today, this is why Yin yoga should always be practiced alongside Yang yoga, the two are opposing sides of the same coin and both are needed to obtain true balance in your life.

The position should be moved into slowly, it should encourage you to be still and in touch with your inner self and to hold the position for a long period of time. Finally, you should release the pose slowly to ensure no harm is done to the body or mind.

The ancient Chinese believed that Yin yoga was a method of controlling and connecting with the qi energy that is present in every living being. This energy is present in everything that you do, it comes in and out of the body in the same way as you breathe and is an essential companion to yin and yang. Yin yoga and Yang yoga are both ways in which you can get in touch with the qi energy in your body and, by listening to the stillness learn to understand the needs of your body and direct your energy accordingly. Balance is the key principle of yoga, the rise of Yin yoga can be said to be an effect of too much Yang yoga. The two must be balanced to ensure everything is harmonious. Yoga studios around the western world now generally offer both Yin and Yang yoga classes; it is recommended to study both disciplines.

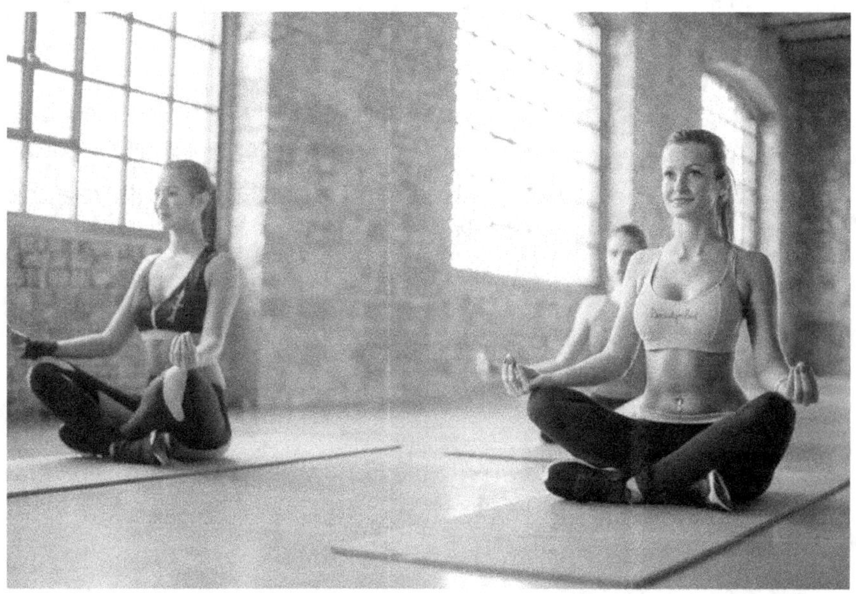

Yin yoga can, in theory, be practiced anywhere. Certainly, the guiding principle of Yin yoga advocates that there are no absolutes, only what is best for each person. However, to ensure you make the most of the time you have available it is best to follow these guidelines:

- Find a space where you are unlikely to be disturbed. This will mean away from other people and the background noise that comes with them. Of course, the better you become at Yin yoga and focusing your attention inwards the easier it will be to block out external events. You may also find it beneficial, when first starting Yin yoga, to have your back to any window or potential distraction.

- Ideally Yin yoga should be practiced when your muscles are cold; this is to ensure that the exercises work on the connective tissues and not the muscles. Cold muscles will pass on the stress to the connective tissues easier than warm muscles will.

- Your muscles will be colder first thing in the morning as they have not had the opportunity to warm up by completing any exercises. This makes first thing a good time to perform your Yin yoga exercises.

- Last thing at night can also be a good time to do your exercises. This will not provide as much of a benefit to your muscles as they will be warmer from the day's activities. However, Yin yoga is very relaxing, and this can be of great benefit to the mind and body at the end of a stressful day.

- Yin yoga can also be a great way to warm up before a more strenuous Yang yoga session. It will not only warm your muscles and stretch both them and the connecting tissues; it will also ensure you are in the right frame of mind for your Yang exercises.

- Yin yoga is very important in spring and summer as these tend to be much more hectic times of year. As such, it is particularly important to create an exercise regime and stick to it. This will ensure you stay balanced and focused.

- Equally, if you find that your life has become very busy and even more stressful than normal it will be essential to make extra time for your Yin yoga. It is during the busiest times in your life that yoga can often be overlooked, yet this is actually when it is most important; it will prevent you from becoming over stressed.

- You may have noticed that travelling is very tiring, whether walking, driving flying or even using the train. This is because, despite most of the time being spent sat, it is actually a yang activity. Finding the time to do some Yin yoga after a trip will help to rebalance your body and rebuild your energy levels.

There are also general guidelines which should be considered before you undertake Yin yoga, even though it is less strenuous than Yang yoga or many other exercises:

- Being pregnant does not mean you cannot practice Yin yoga. It does, however, mean that you should check with your doctor to ensure it is safe for you and your unborn baby.

- If you already have a health condition, such as high blood pressure or diabetes it is best to check with a physician before you start any form of yoga.

- Perfume or after-shave should be avoided if you are going to perform yoga. Many of the exercises require deep breathing and it can be potentially harmful breathing in these fumes for an extended period.

- Ideally you should not eat within two hours of the start of your class or exercise routine.

- Yin yoga is still strenuous, and it is advisable not to do it when you are exhausted. If you really feel the need to do so, keep the exercises short and stick to the gentler positions.

- Prolonged exposure to the sun will deplete the body's reserves and may leave you at risk of dehydration. If you have spent a long time in the sun it is better to avoid your Yin yoga practice and allow your body to recover.

- Watches or bracelets can become uncomfortable when you are holding a pose for a long time. It is better to remove them before you start a session; if you wear glasses it is better to remove these as well.

- Loose, comfortable clothing is essential to ensure you can hold your poses for the time intended. Anything restrictive will be an issue!

- As Yin yoga is a passive form of exercise you will not generate much heat internally. It is therefore essential to be prepared for this. You may wish to turn the thermostat up or to add an extra layer or two.

- Equally, you should make sure that the spot your practice in is well away from any drafts or moving cold air; this can quickly lower your body temperature and ruin a good session.

- Cushions and other sorts of padding are essential to ensure you are comfortable in a variety of poses. Equally, it is advisable to have a thick yoga mat. Many of the exercises are completed whilst sitting or lying down so the possibility of losing grip thanks to sweaty hands is not really an option and a thick mat will be adequate; as well as more comfortable.

- Allow yourself enough time. If you know you only have an hour then aim to finish your practice within forty-five minutes. You do not need to be rushed; this will destroy the effects of the exercise and probably stop you from relaxing fully during your session.

Chapter 20.
Yoga Poses

Please note that for each pose, in addition to the props listed, you'll of course need your yoga mat. I also recommend laying a half-fold blanket over your mat for added comfort and keeping another blanket nearby to cover yourself in case you need a little extra warmth. In any of the reclining postures, you may cover your eyes with an eye pillow or small washcloth to help you relax more deeply.

Opening Pose •20 to 30 minutes

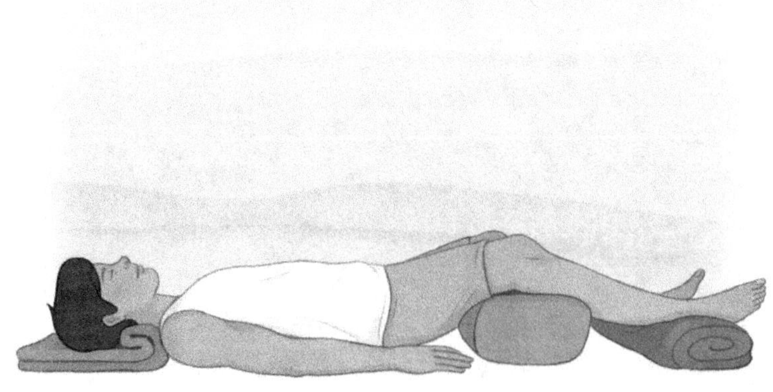

PROPS

Bolster (or 2 rolled blankets or a large pillow)

Blanket roll

Square eighth-fold blanket (or neck pillow)

PRECAUTIONS

- If you are pregnant, substitute Pregnant Goddess or Side Lying Pose.

- If you experience lower back or knee pain, place two blocks under your bolster or roll up three blankets to make a bigger bolster.

BENEFITS

- Maintains and supports the natural curves of your spine.

- Softens your psoas, the deep hip flexor muscles that can become chronically contracted if you spend extended periods sitting, and diaphragm muscle to support a natural, easy breath.

- Relaxes your whole body to aid in stress reduction, slows heart rate, and lowers blood pressure.

- Helps relieve lower back pain.

- Encourages feelings of grounding, belonging, and peace.

INSTRUCTIONS

1. From a sitting position, draw your knees over the bolster and rest your ankles on the blanket roll.

2. Lie back and rest your head on the eighth-fold blanket. Roll up the edge of the blanket so it supports the curve of your neck without forcing your chin toward your chest.

3. Cover yourself with a blanket, cover your eyes, and release your arms alongside your body with your palms facing up.

4. Remain in Basic Relaxation Pose for up to 30 minutes. To exit, draw your knees in toward your chest, roll to one side, and press yourself up to a sitting position.

TIP

Adding weight can help make this pose feel even more grounding. Place a heavy folded blanket or yoga sandbag on your chest or across your lap to help you relax more deeply.

Simple Supported Side Bend

3 to 5 minutes per side

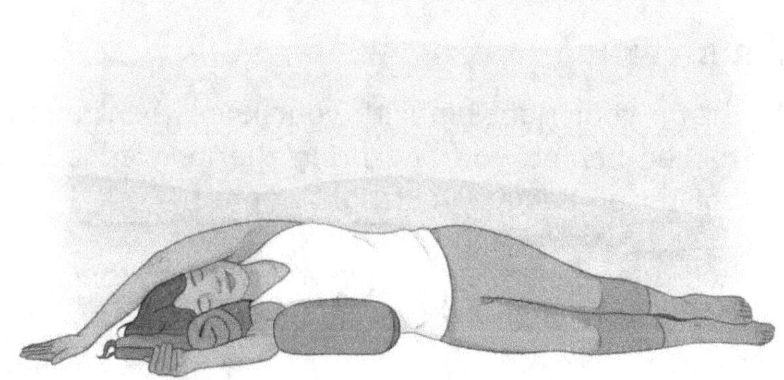

PROPS

Bolster (or 2 rolled blankets or a large pillow)

Square eighth-fold blanket

PRECAUTIONS

- If you have a spinal injury, replace the bolster with one or two stacked long eighth-fold blankets to reduce the curve in your spine.

BENEFITS

- Gently stretches your obliques, latissimus dorsi, and intercostal muscles.

- Gently decompresses your spine.

- Invites your breath to deepen.

- Supports and maintains your spine in normal, healthy lateral flexion.

- Helps relieve lower back pain.

- Encourages a feeling of flexibility.

INSTRUCTIONS

1. Sit on your right hip with your knees bent and feet tucked behind you and bring the long edge of the bolster up against your right thigh.

2. Roll up the blanket and place it on the other side of the bolster with a small gap in between.

3. Lay your right side over the bolster, placing your right shoulder in the gap between the bolster and the blanket. Release your right arm out in front of you and rest your head on the blanket.

4. Rest your left arm on your side or draw it up alongside your left ear for a little more length.

5. Remain in the side bend for 3 to 5 minutes. To exit, place your left hand onto the bolster and press yourself up. Leave the props as they are and turn yourself around to sitting on your left hip to repeat the pose on the other side.

TIP

Place a blanket or pillow between your knees for more support or to relieve discomfort in your knees or hips.

Grounding Spinal Twist

Twist •3 to 5 minutes per side

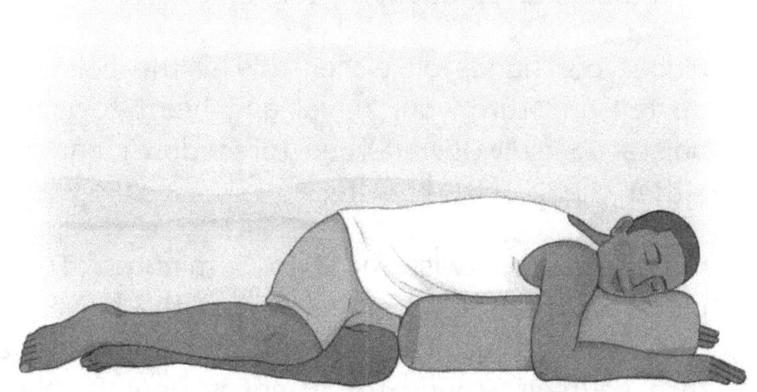

PROPS

Bolster (or 2 rolled blankets or a large pillow)

PRECAUTIONS

- If spinal rotation is contraindicated for you (in the case of spinal injury or pregnancy), skip this pose.

BENEFITS

- Supports and maintains your spine in normal, healthy rotation.

- Gently decompresses your spine.

- Gently stretches your lumbar muscles.

- Helps relieve back pain.

- Invites feelings of connection and stability.

INSTRUCTIONS

1. Sit on your right hip with your knees bent and your feet tucked in behind you and bring the narrow end of the bolster up against your right hip.

2. Place your hands on either side of the bolster. Sit up tall and turn your navel and heart toward the bolster. Slowly lower your torso down and place either cheek on the bolster.

3. Remain in the twist for 3 to 5 minutes. To exit, place your hands on either side of the bolster and press yourself up. Leave the bolster where it is and turn yourself around to sitting on your left hip to repeat the pose on the other side.

TIP

It's common to try to support yourself with your arms in this pose, so make sure to take your elbows a little wider and relax, letting the bolster do the work for you.

Spine Lengthening Pose

Backbend •5 to 10 minutes

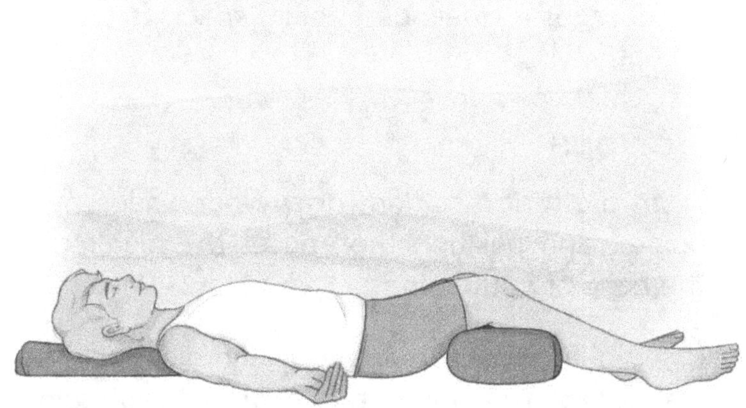

PROPS

Bolster (or 2 rolled blankets or a large pillow)

Blanket roll

PRECAUTIONS

- If you are pregnant, substitute Pregnant Goddess Pose or Supported Heart Pose with Legs Over a Bolster.

BENEFITS

- Gently decompresses your spine.

- Supports and maintains your spine in normal,

healthy extension.

- Gently stretches your chest and shoulders.

- Reverses the effects of long periods spent sitting and slouching.

- Invites your breath to deepen.

- Encourages feelings of spaciousness and receptivity.

INSTRUCTIONS

1. From a sitting position, draw your knees over the bolster and position the end of the blanket roll at the base of your spine.

2. Use your arms for support and lie back so the blanket roll runs along the length of your spine and supports your head.

3. Release your arms alongside you with your palms facing up and relax.

4. Remain in Spine Lengthening Pose for 5 to 10 minutes. To exit, draw your knees in toward your chest, roll to one side, and press yourself up to a sitting position.

TIP

A common error is to sit on the blanket roll before lying down and miss out on the spinal massage in this pose. Make sure your hips are between the bolster and blanket roll before you lie down to create length.

Heart Pose

Backbend •5 to 10 minutes

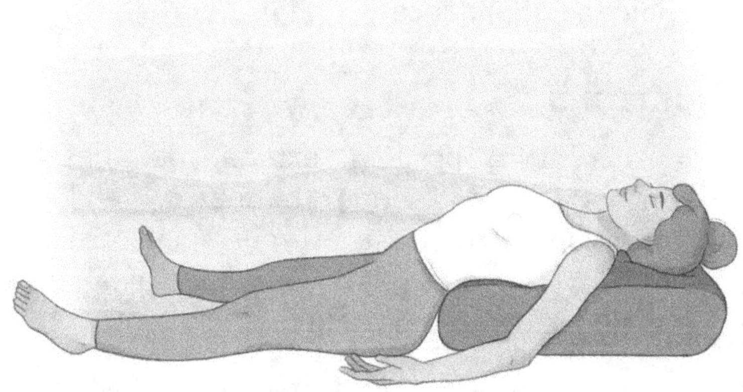

PROPS

Bolster (or 2 rolled blankets or a large pillow)

PRECAUTIONS

- If you are pregnant, substitute Pregnant Goddess Pose.

- If you suffer from lower back pain or sensitivity, substitute Supported Heart Pose with Legs Over a Bolster.

BENEFITS

- Gently decompresses your spine.

- Gently stretches your chest, shoulders, and

abdomen.

- Reverses the effects of long periods spent sitting and slouching.

- Invites your breath to deepen.

- Naturally boosts your energy and supports feelings of joy and abundance.

INSTRUCTIONS

1. From a sitting position, extend your legs out in front of you and bring the narrow end of the bolster up to the base of your spine. Using your arms for support, relax your abdominal muscles and lie back onto the bolster.

2. Remain in Heart Pose for 5 to 10 minutes. To exit, bend your knees, roll to one side, and press yourself up to a sitting position.

TIP

If the bolster feels too high for your spine in this position and the sensation is too intense, move your hips away from the bolster slightly to create some space and lessen the curve in your spine.

Supported Forward Fold

Forward Bend •5 to 8 minutes

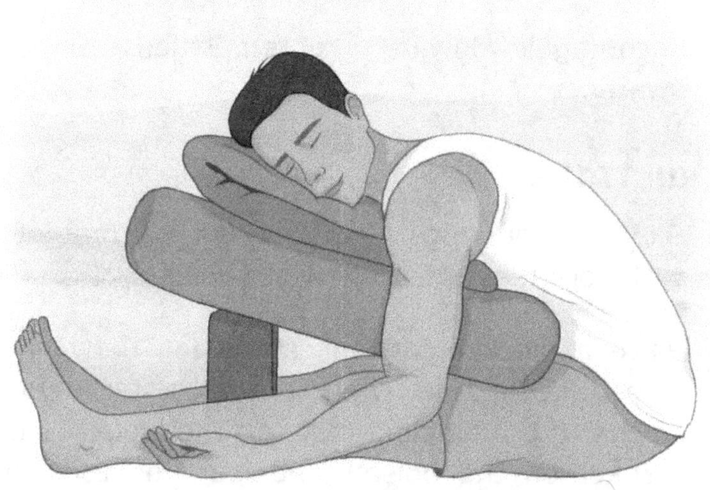

PROPS

Bolster (or 2 rolled blankets or a large pillow)

Block (or large hardcover book)

Square eighth-fold blanket

PRECAUTIONS

- If forward bending is contraindicated for your spine, substitute Legs Up the Wall or Head to Bolster Pose.

BENEFITS

- Supports and maintains your spine in normal,

healthy flexion.

- Gently stretches your back muscles and hamstrings.

- Can help relieve neck and jaw tension and headache.

- Encourages inward contemplation and self-awareness.

INSTRUCTIONS

1. Sit with your legs stretched out in front of you, with your feet about hip-width apart.

2. Place a block on its tallest setting between your shins. Set the narrow end of the bolster in your lap so that the other end rests on the block. Place the blanket on the bolster and lean forward, resting your abdomen, heart, and cheek on the bolster. Relax your arms by your sides.

3. Halfway through, turn your head and place the opposite cheek down for an equal stretch of your neck.

4. Remain in Supported Forward Fold for 5 to 8 minutes. To exit, press your hands into the bolster and sit up.

TIP

If you can't easily bring your torso to the bolster, add more blankets to bring the bolster to you so you can relax in the pose.

Supported Child's Pose

Forward Bend •5 to 8 minutes

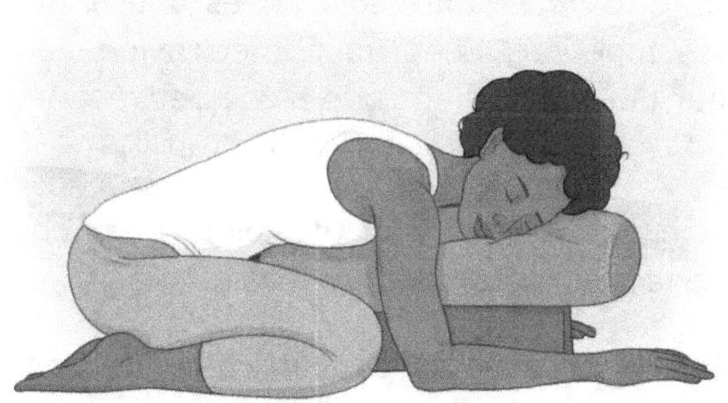

PROPS

Bolster (or 2 rolled blankets or a large pillow)

2 blocks (or large hardcover books)

PRECAUTIONS

- If you are unable to bend your knees enough to support this pose, substitute Supported Forward Fold or Supported Half Frog.

BENEFITS

- Supports and maintains your spine in normal, healthy flexion.

- Gently stretches your back muscles, glutes, and quadriceps muscles.

- Helps relieve back pain.

- Helps soothe anxiety and restlessness.

- Fosters a sense of calm and steadiness.

INSTRUCTIONS

1. Come to your hands and knees and bring your big toes together. Keep your knees wide. Sit back on your heels and place one block between your knees and the other block just in front of it.

2. Place the bolster on the blocks so one end is between your knees.

3. Using your arms for support, bow forward onto the bolster and place your abdomen, heart, and either cheek on the bolster. Relax your arms.

4. Halfway through, turn your head and place the opposite cheek down for an equal stretch of your neck.

5. Remain in Supported Child's Pose for 5 to 8 minutes. To exit the pose, place your palms down on either side of the bolster and press down to lift to sitting on your heels. Come onto your seat and stretch out your legs.

TIP

If your hips don't come all the way to your heels or you feel strain in your knees here, place folded blankets in the back of your knees for support.

Reclining Butterfly

Hip Opener •5 to 8 minutes

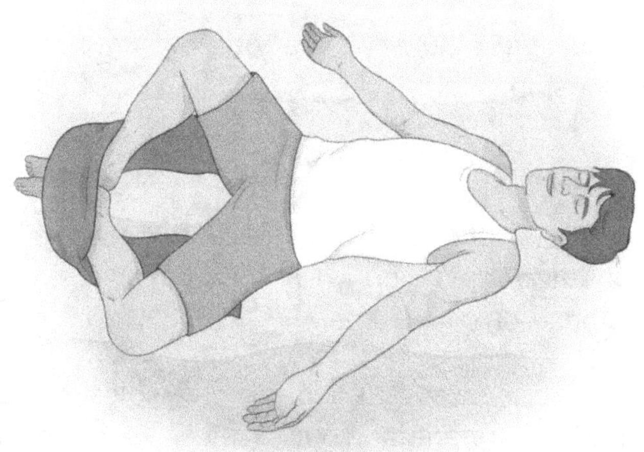

PROPS

Long eighth-fold blanket

Blanket roll

PRECAUTIONS

- If you are pregnant, substitute Pregnant Goddess Pose.

- If you experience discomfort in your knees or hips in this pose, use blocks or more blankets to prop up your thighs.

BENEFITS

- Supports and maintains your hips in gentle, healthy

external rotation.

- Gently stretches your inner thigh muscles.

- Helps relieve hip pain due to long periods spent sitting.

- Encourages dual sensations of grounding and expansion.

INSTRUCTIONS

1. From a sitting position, place the long eighth-fold blanket behind you with the narrow end touching the base of your spine.

2. Bend your knees and bring the soles of your feet together, opening your knees wide to make a diamond shape with your legs.

3. Place the middle of the blanket roll on top of your feet, then draw the ends around your ankles to meet behind your heels so your outer shins are supported.

4. Using your hands for support, lie back onto the blanket behind you.

5. Remain in Reclining Butterfly for 5 to 8 minutes. To exit, use your hands to draw your knees together, then roll to one side and press yourself up to a sitting position.

TIP

If you've been feeling down or sitting a lot and want to increase feelings of openness, take your arms out wide. If you've been feeling scattered or anxious and are seeking more grounding, place one hand on your heart and the other on your abdomen.

Elevated Legs Up the Wall

Inversion •5 to 10 minutes

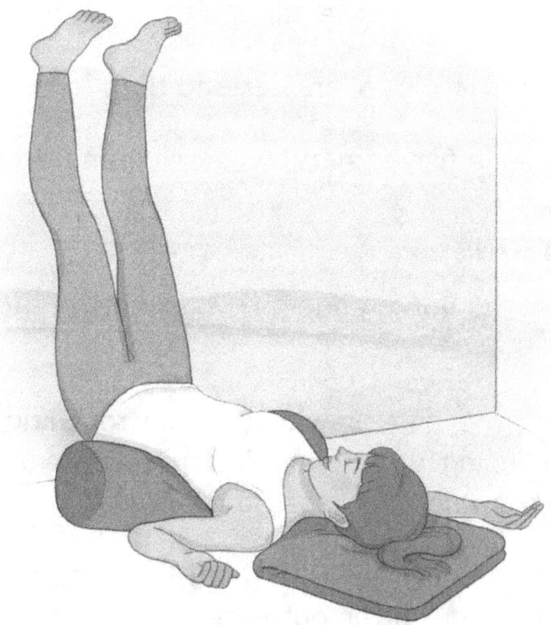

PROPS

Bolster (or 2 rolled blankets or a large pillow)

Square eighth-fold blanket

PRECAUTIONS

- Inverting is contraindicated for pregnancy, hernia, severe acid reflux, brain injuries, glaucoma, and high blood pressure. In these cases, substitute Legs Up the Bolster.

- If this pose aggravates your lower back, substitute Legs Up the Wall.

BENEFITS

- Supports your body in a gentle inversion, taking gravitational pressure off your legs and feet.

- Improves heart rate variability.

- Can alleviate swollen feet and tired legs.

- Soothes a frayed nervous system and tired mind.

INSTRUCTIONS

1. Place the long edge of your bolster against the wall.

2. Sit on the bolster with one hip touching the wall; then, using your arms for support, lean back and gently swing your legs up the wall.

3. Lie back and use the blanket to support your head. Release your arms out wide.

4. Remain in Elevated Legs Up the Wall for 5 to 10 minutes. To exit, bend your knees into your chest and carefully roll off the bolster to one side, then press yourself up to a sitting position.

TIP

If you've spent a long day on your feet, try this pose right before bed to relieve aches and pains in your legs and feet and calm your mind to prepare for a good night's sleep.

Chapter 21.
Navigating Chakra Yoga

Approach the chakra yoga practice by first discovering where your blockages are, and then learning which poses and sequences balance the chakra that you need to work on. This will help inform your practice and give you a guided and structured approach that will be more effective in healing you faster. Once you have decided what you would like to focus on, put a plan into place that will help you work toward achieving your goals.

Also, be aware that as you become more in touch with your body, you may notice imbalances in multiple chakras. You might want to work on everything at once but be cautious. As with most things, it is best to focus on one thing at a time. You may move through a yoga sequence that addresses different chakras, giving you a full-body experience; however, if you have a specific goal of unlocking your root chakra, for instance, then start with that and focus most of your energy there first.

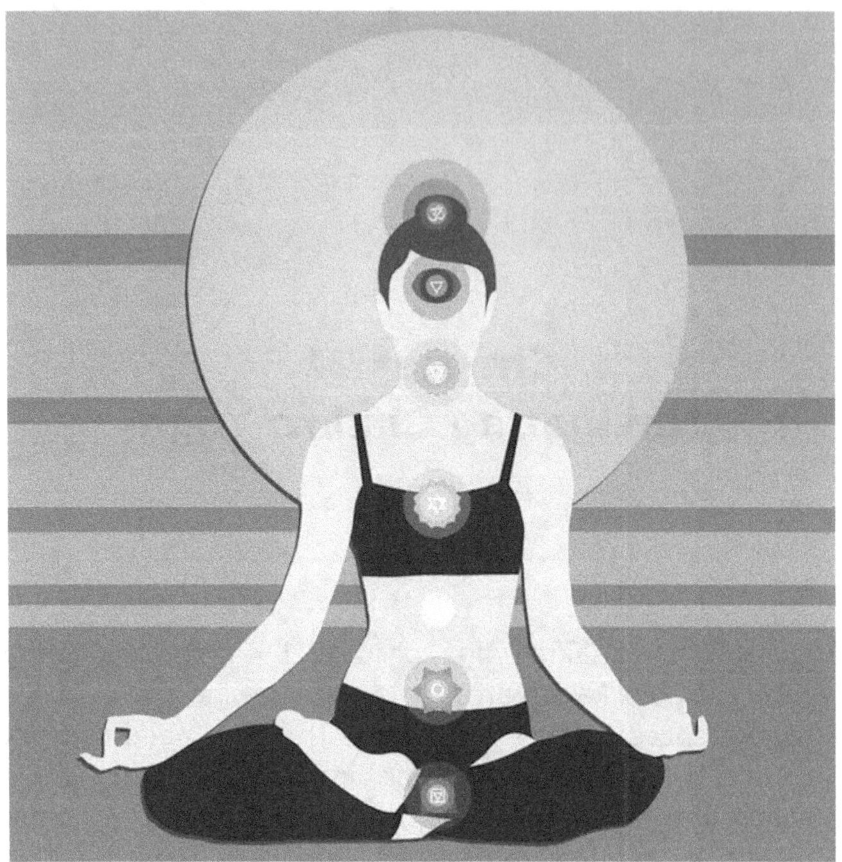

There are seven major chakras. The root chakra is known as the first major chakra because it is at the bottom of the spine and acts as the foundation for the rest of the chakras. If you are looking to balance more than one of your chakras, it is best to begin at the lowest one. This will create a ripple effect as healing works its way up the system along the spine, building a solid foundation for all the chakras to heal and thrive.

Practice as often as you can, but at least once a week. If you can practice daily, go for it. Start with one session and try to fit more into your schedule as time goes on. You will likely find yourself wanting to increase the frequency of your sessions because of how good you feel afterward.

Creating Your Own Practice

Since you are reading this book, it is likely that you are looking to form an at-home yoga practice and ritual for yourself. Creating a dedicated yoga space in your home is a great way to generate habit and a sense of desire to get onto your mat and practice regularly. This space should be aesthetically pleasing to you and calming for your mind. It should help the flow of creativity and inspire you not only in your yoga practice, but in other areas of your life as well. If you do not have a designated space in your home where you can keep your yoga props out at all times, store them, and when you take them out for practice, you are creating a ritual—a tradition—that you will ultimately find a regular sense of comfort in.

I will go into the necessary yoga props in a bit more detail later, but first I'll mention that it is really nice to have a dedicated yoga mat that is only yours. This yoga mat is your sacred place, where you can come to heal your mind, body, and spirit. It should be treated well, cleaned, and stored in a protective way. It is also common for people to use the public mats at their studio or gym where they attend classes. While this is a fine option if you are short on space at home, it is not ideal if you are looking to build a personal chakra yoga practice for yourself and your overall healing. I highly encourage you to invest in and take good care of your own yoga mat for your practice.

As you begin to develop your own practice, you will come to find that your yoga mat is your special zone, an area that brings you joy. I have had the same yoga mat for about five years, and it is still going strong. The dusty pink color brings me joy every time I look at it, and the material feels good when it meets my skin. I have great affinity for my mat, and I almost think of it as an old friend who is always there for me no matter what is going on in my life. I believe that everyone should have the same kind of relationship with their yoga mat because it strengthens the special bond you have with your yoga practice.

Speaking of bonding with your practice: It is important to not only set up a designated yoga space, but also to establish a routine for yourself. Consider what you would like to accomplish and use that as motivation to keep coming back to your practice. Goal setting—to have a clear picture in your mind about what you would like to achieve—is so important in all aspects of life, and your yoga practice is no different. Goals will help you establish your practice on your own terms and stay motivated to keep coming back to your mat.

LISTENING TO YOUR BODY

This book will guide you step-by-step through the yoga poses and sequences to take the guesswork out of what you should be doing when practicing the yoga asanas. This will aid your practice, but it is no substitute for an in-person yoga teacher and your knowledge about your own body. If you find yourself struggling, or if something does not feel good, then move out of that pose; do not force yourself. Use modifications and yoga props where needed to help the pose feel better in your body. Always use your body as a guide and listen to its cues. While it is great to challenge yourself to grow and improve, forcing yourself into a yoga pose that you are not ready for is never the answer. There are ways to work your way up to achieving the full expression of the poses, and you must be patient with yourself.

It is important to recognize the difference between the good type of pain, which is helping you get stronger, and the bad type of pain, which is causing your body harm. If you experience sharp pain in a joint (where two bones are fitted together), then move out of the pose immediately. Dull pain in the middle of the muscles is okay as your muscles stretch and gain flexibility. Your body is very smart, and you can trust its signals. You just have to know how to interpret the messages.

Holding Poses

In this book, I will advise a suggested amount of time to hold each pose within a sequence, but it is also important to listen to your body and make that decision for yourself. As you deepen your practice and get more accustomed to practicing yoga regularly, you will begin to develop an intuition about how long to stay in each pose.

For a hatha or vinyasa yoga class, you should hold the poses for three to five deep and full breaths, in and out through the nose. For a yin or restorative practice, you will hold the poses for much longer, generally three to five minutes each, which translates to 20 to 30 deep and full breaths. But these are not hard-and-fast rules. At times, your teacher or the yoga sequence you are following may advise you to hold a certain pose for a bit longer to emphasize a certain movement, or they may just pass through a pose more quickly. It depends on many different factors, including the class style, the purpose or theme of that class or sequence, and the teacher.

You can also look for signals from your body to let you know when it is time to exit a pose. As I mentioned earlier, you will need to listen to your body and understand which types of pain are good and which are bad. Your body will always want to choose the path of least resistance, so understanding that some types of pain are good is crucial to your growth. When in doubt, if the pain is too intense, come out of it until you have a better grasp on what you should and should not be feeling. This wisdom will come over time, so as always, be patient with yourself and continue to practice regularly and consistently.

LEAVING YOUR COMFORT ZONE

Many people in the yoga world speak about finding your "edge" in the pose and taking your body there before coming out of it. You will learn more about where your personal edge is over time as you progress through your yoga practice. A good guideline for finding where that edge is for yourself is understanding when your body's survival mode tends to kick in. This is the moment when your body generally gets tired and wants to choose the path of least resistance. Once you realize that the pain or discomfort you may be experiencing is not the bad type of pain and you are able to stay in the pose without causing harm to your body, then you can acknowledge and move past your edge.

When you reach and move past your edge, not only does your body improve, get stronger, and gain flexibility, but you also experience the change of energy flow within your chakras. Change must occur in order to achieve balance in your chakras, especially if you have a blockage in a certain area. You will learn this over time through your personal journey, so trust the process and be patient with yourself.

Harnessing Your Breath

The breath is a vital aspect of a yoga practice and moving through the yoga poses, and it can also be used as a tool to support and advance your practice. There are specific breathing techniques and exercises that you can do to feel relaxed, gain energy, feel grounded, and more. However, you can simply incorporate breathing into your asana practice as well to help you feel better in the poses and improve within your body.

The life force of your body is your breath, and therefore "prana," "breath," and "energy" can be used interchangeably. While there is a difference between energy and breath in terms of physicality and location within the body, breath is simply the release or intake of energy. When you inhale, you are bringing energy and power in, and that energy continues to flow through the body and the chakras. When you exhale, you are releasing energy out of the body, continuing the pathway of the flow of energy.

Breath can be used as a tool to help you feel more relaxed and slow down your heart rate if you are feeling anxious. It can also be used to deepen a stretch. As you exhale, you can gently ease your body a bit deeper into the stretch, coming to your edge and continuing to breathe through any discomfort. You can also use your breath to connect to your subconscious during meditation. The act of focusing on your breath brings your attention to what is happening inside your body and allows you to observe how you are feeling on the inside. As you get to know yourself and your body on a deeper level, you will also build a deeper relationship with your breath and gain a greater understanding of it.

GRANTHIS (KNOTS)

Granthi translates to "knot," and it refers to the concept that blocked energy is restrictive and difficult to untie. If you find that you have blocked chakras, you will likely be dealing with granthis. These restrict the passage of prana throughout the body and can be caused by a variety of happenings in your life. They result in you becoming stuck in your ways, not allowing yourself to be open to new possibilities. These can be general or more specific, depending on the area where the granthi exists and what caused it. There are ways to release your granthis that are detailed later, and you can incorporate them into your chakra yoga practice.

BANDHAS (LOCKS)

Practicing the bandhas ("locks") can help in releasing your granthis and aid in your quest to unblock your chakras. Bandhas help you shift and move your prana to different areas of the body where your granthis and chakra blocks may be restricting its access. There are four bandhas in the body that you can incorporate into your chakra yoga practice:

1. Mula Bandha. This is the root lock, and to execute it, you must activate and squeeze in the muscles in the perineum area at the first chakra, Muladhara. This is commonly known as a Kegel, and it is often practiced strengthening vaginal muscles before and after childbirth.

2. Uddiyana Bandha. This lock happens in your

abdominal area, and it is the act of drawing all the organs in your abdomen upward as you bend forward. You can rest your hands on your legs as you are bringing those muscles and organs up and in.

3. Jalandhara Bandha. This lock takes place in the neck area, and it can be done by sitting up tall in a cross-legged position with your hands on your legs. Draw your sternum up and your chin down to a place where they meet each other halfway.

Practicing these bandhas and holding them for as long as you are able to will make you stronger and aid in the flow of energy throughout the body.

RELEASING YOUR PAST

At times, as we begin to open and balance our chakras, many past traumas and tensions can get brought to the forefront. As humans, we often suppress traumatic and painful experiences that have happened in our past to avoid feeling the pain. As I mentioned before, our minds and bodies usually choose the path of least resistance, and sometimes avoiding emotional pain is a part of that path.

While it may be more comfortable to avoid pain, it is important to lean into it and push through so we can get past it and move on. If this happens to you during your chakra yoga practice, sit with whatever feelings come up for you and observe them. If you need to cry, it is absolutely okay. Do not be afraid to let it out and release whatever you are feeling. You can even incorporate journaling about the experience, which often helps get the thoughts and feelings out.

Once you observe your thoughts and feelings, acknowledge that whatever you're pulling up is not happening now; it is just a memory. Also acknowledge that your thoughts are not you, they do not define you, and you can observe them without judgment before you watch them fade away. It may take a bit of time to feel better, but you must not repress those feelings again once they resurface. Be sure to take the time to release them properly and work through them by way of observation, journaling, and emotional release before moving forward.

Chapter 22.
Yoga Techniques

It is finally time to talk about the four particular techniques I use to personalize individual Yoga practices. Now is the time to progress at a rapid pace!

Once we have chosen a style of Yoga that we feel fits us well, it is time to learn how to get even more out of it. All these techniques can be applied to any Yoga class you attend, whether at a studio learning from a teacher or at home using a DVD or podcast.

The first two techniques are geared toward increasing flexibility, the second two are geared toward increasing strength. It is imperative that you find a synergistic balance between the two. When you feel that you are comfortable with the techniques, you can begin to apply them to other areas of your life as well.

At the end of each technique description, I include a story about one of my actual students, and how that particular technique helped them with his or her unique situation. It is my hope that these anecdotes will shed some light on some of the real-life conundrums we all face.

Technique #1

Breathe and Sink

This involves proper adaptation of Proprioceptive Neuromuscular Facilitation (PNF).

Yes, I know. Big words!

This is the scientific backing for why it is necessary to practice Yoga at least twice per week. PNF is what triggers a muscle to relax and release. When PNF is properly activated, it lasts for up to 72 hours. Meaning, when you trigger that amount of flexibility in your muscle, it will remain that flexible for up to 72 hours.

When practiced, the results are pretty astonishing. This procedure was taught to me by one of my teachers (whom I respect very much). This teacher is also a physical therapist. It is pretty simple: when you stretch, every time you exhale, allow your body to sink deeper into the stretch.

This process 'tricks' the muscles into relaxing and then, in turn, releasing. If your muscles can relax long enough to allow oxygen to integrate into them and start to flow, then they can safely allow the flexibility to increase every time.

Now, when we practice our physical Yoga postures, we are practicing many forms of PNF using our own body weight. If you have done the math in your head, you now understand why it is important to practice Yoga at least twice per week. The increase in flexibility lasts for 72 hours, so you need to utilize PNF by doing Yoga at least this often. This is how you will rapidly gain and maintain the flexibility in your muscles.

The best way to consciously apply PNF through your Yoga practice is to make sure to sink a little deeper into each pose that requires muscular extension with each exhalation.

For example, if you are in a forward bend, every time you exhale, allow the weight of your body to make your torso sink even closer to your legs. The longer you hold a pose, the closer your torso will get to your legs, and the more you are going to get out of it.

Now, PNF is more difficult to apply to some poses, such as push-up positions or standing postures. But it is possible if you use mindfulness to observe which muscles are actually activated when you do them. But this will only come with practice and observance.

If this seems like too much for you, don't worry. Just use this technique when you do poses that focus on stretching more than strengthening. Like a seated forward fold or a side bend or twist. You want to safely increase your flexibility without over stretching the muscles and causing them to be strained and flimsy.

Hot Yoga can speed up this process quite a bit. But we also need to be careful not to soften up the muscles or the ligaments to the point we can pull them. This is how pregnant women can damage themselves because, during pregnancy, women's ligaments become more malleable. This leads to increased flexibility but also increased risk of injury. Also, warming up the muscles too much can lead to inflammation and deterioration of the tissue if the muscles don't already have a strong foundation of freely flowing oxygen and decent blood flow.

But as long as you mindfully and consciously practice PNF during a hot Yoga class, then you will avoid injury due to over stretching and over warming. We will talk more about hot Yoga later in this book.

My primary goal as a Yoga instructor is to teach people how to properly take care of their bodies. To help them understand their forms are unique and then help them learn to adjust their attitudes and physical practices accordingly.

Another helpful benefit of PNF is that it breaks up buildups of connective tissue, which we will talk about in the next technique.

Tyler's Story

Tyler wandered into one of my group Yoga classes one day in the summertime when we were practicing outside in the park. The class was entirely donation based, so it was open to anyone who wanted to join us. He arrived late and didn't have a mat, so he just tried to follow along with the others in the grass.

After the class, I approached him to thank him for coming and to ask some questions about what brought him there. He told me he used to see the class practicing in the mornings when he would run by on his way to the gym. He was a 26-year-old Caucasian and quite the athlete. A bodybuilder, rock climber, and runner who also competed in triathlons.

But a few months earlier, he had started having serious pain in his lower back and joints. His athletic lifestyle had begun to turn against him. He kept seeing all these people practicing Yoga in the park together, many of them much older than he was, and he decided they were onto something. So, he came to check it out.

I had watched him struggle through the unfamiliar poses while he tried to keep up with the others. He said it was quite the reality check for him not to be able to keep up with all these people who were double and triple his age. I told him I would be able to help him if he would consider one-on-one classes.

He agreed, and we started working together that week.

Just as I had suspected, Tyler's biggest problem was his lack of flexibility. He spent all his training time on cardio and strength building. His muscles were certainly strong and bulky; so much so, in fact, that everything had tightened up around his nerves, causing nerves and muscles to spasm.

We worked together for about six months, applying all my techniques but focusing heavily on Technique #1. PNF. He was a very shallow breather, which is common in athletes of his stature. But with time, I taught him to breathe deep into his belly rather than shallow breaths in the chest.

Once he became more comfortable with how to perform the postures, and how to use the exhalation to deepen them, I suggested he try Bikram Yoga.

With that, he had found his Yoga-soulmate!

Bikram Yoga proved to be a fantastic compliment to his athletic lifestyle. He told me that applying the Breath and Sink method I had showed him allowed him to relax in the postures enough to let his body surrender to the benefits.

In a short amount of time, his pain subsided completely, and he was competing in triathlons once again. He is still attending Bikram Yoga classes no less than twice a week (as I suggested for full PNF benefits), and recently told me he has convinced many of his friends to join him as well.

Technique #2

Breaking Up the Fuzz

This technique will not be as easy to apply in a group Yoga classroom as it will when you are at home. This is because it will require you to hold the poses longer. If you are at home practicing alone on your mat, or in front of a DVD, you can simply pause in each of the seated or reclining poses. Stay there for a minimum of 10 to 25 breaths. With each exhalation, see if you can stretch a little bit deeper into the pose.

I am now going to share with you the connective tissue story I tell all my students at some point in our time together. The teacher in my Yoga Anatomy training course called a buildup of connective tissue "The Fuzz."

Every night when you sleep, or whenever your body isn't mobile for that matter, your muscles and joints begin to develop a thin layer of the Fuzz. This is a white, sticky material that does indeed look quite fuzzy. It is really called connective tissue or fascia.

When you wake up in the morning, you stretch yourself out and begin to move around. This breaks up the Fuzz that has built up in your body overnight. The Fuzz is always developing, but if you make a continuous effort to break it apart, all that will remain is a thin layer.

However, if you don't make a continuous effort to break up the Fuzz, it will build up. It will build layer upon layer as if you were adding multiple coats of paint to a surface.

As the layers build up, they become less malleable and begin to calcify. The Fuzz becomes tougher and tougher, and eventually, even hard. Once it reaches this state, it becomes significantly more difficult to break apart.

It is similar to maintaining dental hygiene, where the plaque that builds up on your teeth daily eventually becomes tartar if it is neglected.

If you want to avoid having connective tissue buildup, you need to make sure you are allowing oxygen to flow into your muscles. (Too much connective tissue can suffocate the muscle, leading to muscle atrophy). This is where Yoga comes in.

I had read quite a bit about connective tissue in my other anatomy and Yoga training courses, but I didn't fully understand its significance until I attended an autopsy demonstration on two human cadavers.

The first one was a young and physically fit marathon runner. He had passed away from a head injury, but he had been very active with a good diet and maintained good flexibility and mobility in all his joints.

The second was an elderly woman who had been confined to a wheelchair for the last several decades of her life.

There were several striking differences between their

spines (if you are extremely squeamish or uncomfortable with this topic, I recommend you skip the next two paragraphs).

The young man's spine looked exactly the way one would expect a spine to look. There was a little bit of white, fuzzy-looking stuff around his spine and muscles, but when the instructor ran his finger over it, it broke apart and disintegrated.

The woman's spine, however, looked as if she had years and years of spiderweb buildup wrapped around it as well as all the connecting muscles. It created a thick whitish coating that made the individual vertebrae underneath completely indistinguishable from one another. It was also rock hard to the touch. In fact, the only way to break it apart was to cut it apart with a scalpel and pliers!

I realize this is a very extreme example, but the point is, years and years of neglect can cause serious damage to our bodies.

Now the secret to avoiding this is very simple: move!

Moving and stretching breaks up the Fuzz. If you break it up every day, it won't build up. Therefore, it won't calcify.

But what if this has already started to happen?

Don't worry. It is still reversible. These particular styles are extremely effective in increasing flexibility. This is because you hold the postures for so long. Traditionally, in Yin Yoga, you hold a pose for no less than five minutes, and sometimes as long as 30 minutes!

When you hold a posture for this long, PNF will naturally

take place. But it is always a good idea to be conscious of PNF while doing it to help the process along.

The longer you hold a pose, the deeper your body will go into it. The first Yin Yoga class I attended was pretty life changing. I left feeling like a bowl full of wet spaghetti. My whole body was so relaxed it felt as if I was floating on a cloud as I walked out of the studio.

By actively breaking up my connective tissue, I got myself into poses I never would have dreamed were possible, and that was only my first class! I went once per week, and my flexibility didn't dissipate. This, however, was before I found out that one could be too flexible.

Juan's Story

When I met Juan, he was in his late seventies and had been coming to Yoga classes for about a decade. He was an absolutely delightful Hispanic man with a very thick accent. After his wife died 11 years prior, he started coming to Yoga classes because he had read it could be healing.

Because he was a reasonably healthy man who remained pretty active, he certainly looked younger than he was. He attended our donation-based Yoga classes about five times a week.

What initially caught my interest about his practice was his rounded back and tight, hunched shoulders. When he attempted poses that involved chest and shoulder opening, he was unable to perform them in a way that would be beneficial to his body. When I taught, I would try to help him open up in the pose, but he wasn't really getting it.

I tried to work with him after each class as well, but he clearly needed more time. So, I asked if he would consider one-on-one classes. He seemed a little embarrassed, but he agreed. I reassured him that he wasn't actually doing anything wrong. He was doing a wonderful thing for his body by coming to these Yoga classes so often. The reason I wanted to work with him was because I knew if I could teach him how to open up his upper body, he would get a lot more out of his Yoga practice.

I told him it would take somewhere between three and 12 private lessons to help him get where he needed to be.

Well, he progressed faster than I ever could have imagined!

Once I explained the concept of connective tissue to him and told him the story about the Fuzz, a light bulb seemed to go off above his head.

I spent three lessons showing him how to properly open up his shoulders and chest and sent him back out into the world. I suggested he try some Yin Yoga classes a nearby studio offered, and he reported back to me that he was astonished by how different his body felt.

He had never realized how closed off to the world he felt until he learned how to open himself up. He said that not only did he feel different physically, but he felt emotionally ready to approach the world with an open heart.

He still attends his regular group Yoga classes five times per week, but also, now goes to a Yin Yoga class about once per month in addition. I have literally watched his entire stature evolve since then. He stands up straighter and holds his shoulders back. He even moves with more confidence.

I believe he conquered the Fuzz!

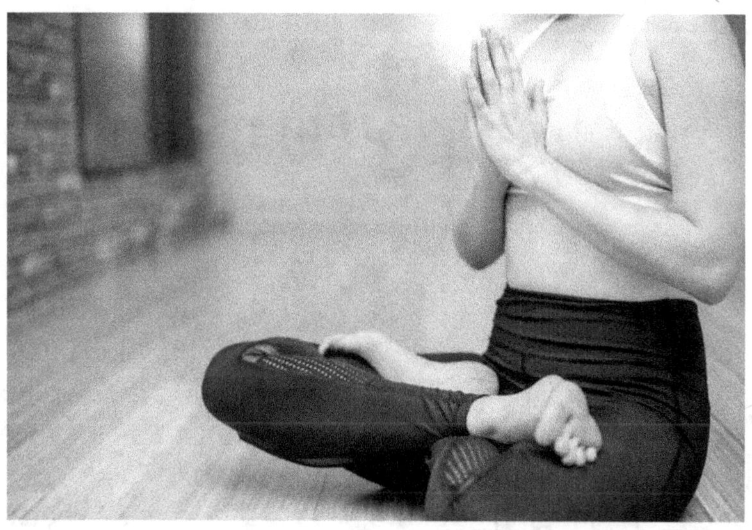

Chapter 23.
Yoga Nidra

Yoga Nidra means "the yoga of sleep," but don't let the name fool you. In truth, this ancient practice is more about learning to wake up. Nidra refers to that daydream state between wakefulness and sleep. Think of the paradox of sleeping wakefulness as a bridge between otherwise disparate elements, such as consciousness and unconsciousness, spirit and form, and the ego-self and the True Self.

Yoga Nidra is essentially a guided meditation during which the practitioner usually lies down, closes their eyes, and becomes very relaxed as they are guided by a facilitator into deeper and deeper layers of relaxed Awareness. By recording the scripts in this book and playing them back, you will be both the facilitator and the practitioner.

A Yoga Nidra practice often lasts between 10 and 45 minutes, during which time the facilitator guides the practitioner systematically into a focused but neutral observation of the five koshas (or sheaths, which you can think of as layers over your True Self). These are the objects of the ego as well as physical sensations, thoughts, and emotions. The method's aim is to help you learn to stop identifying with the ego-self by peeling back the koshas like layers of skin off an onion and instead identify with the core of your True Nature—pure Awareness. It's like napping your way to enlightenment!

While not everyone emerges from every practice having "seen the light," it's incredible how many people report experiencing massive benefits, even after their first session. Rather than tell my students the benefits of the practice, I allow the practice to speak for itself. I typically start a Yoga Nidra class by asking return students how they benefit from the practice. Eager hands shoot into the air as students happily report a wide array of benefits, including lowered stress, being less reactive, greater happiness, better sleep, lowered blood pressure, less anxiety and depression, more energy, accelerated learning, increased creativity, higher performance and productivity, general well-being, better digestion, greater optimism, spiritual insight, confidence, and a grounded sense of purpose, clarity, and optimism.

In more extreme cases, I've personally used Yoga Nidra, often in tandem with a licensed clinical therapist, as a powerful tool to help people who suffer from issues like PTSD, trauma, sexual abuse, chronic anxiety and depression, eating disorders, alcohol and chemical dependency, and chronic and terminal illnesses better cope with their issues. I have also used Yoga Nidra to maximize the performance of world-class artists, including the cast of the Broadway show STOMP, Justin Timberlake's dancers and backup singers, and the dancers of Ballet West. I've trained top-level athletes to use Yoga Nidra to help them perform and win ultramarathons, ultra-cycling events, and Olympic events.

I've even trained high school kids to use Yoga Nidra to conquer test anxiety. At one of my recent trainings, I taught a marriage and family lawyer how to use Yoga Nidra with her clients to help them manage divorce proceedings as calmly and civilly as possible.

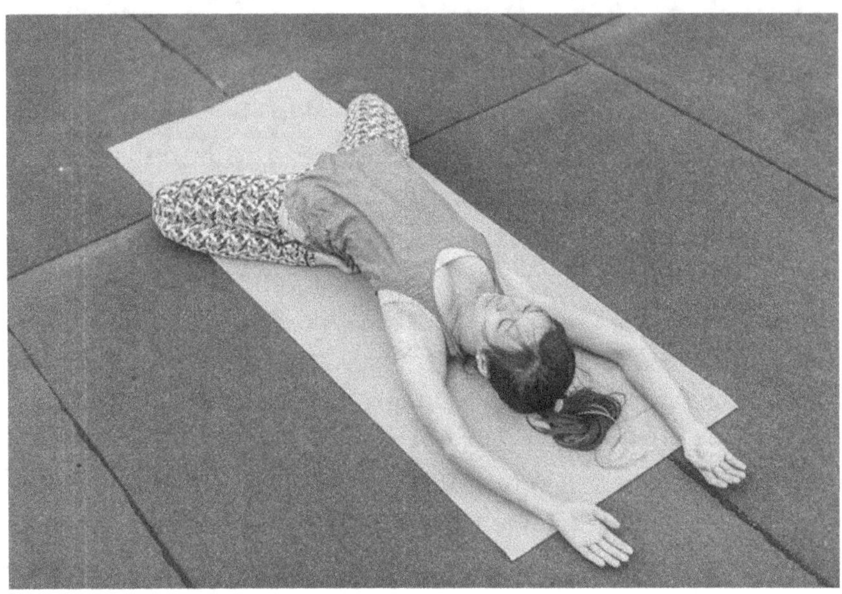

The benefits of Yoga Nidra have also been tested in clinical studies. Currently, Yoga Nidra teachers, such as clinical psychologist Dr. Richard C. Miller, are conducting scientific studies to show how it can benefit war veterans in prisons and hospitals. A report in the Journal of Caring Sciences shows Yoga Nidra to be a successful therapy to help with anxiety, depression, positive well-being, general health, and vitality scores as well as hormonal levels associated with menstrual irregularity.

So how can a practice of simply lying down and being guided through something like a body scan or an examination of your thoughts provoke such remarkable benefits? The idea is that when you're aligned with your

True Self through—and as—deep Awareness, you experience the part of you that is always perfect. More simply, as you experience yourself as Awareness, you experience wholeness. In such wholeness, there's nothing you can't do or be. Wholeness means healed. All the benefits my students call out in class are merely the by-products of wholeness.

One of the essential truths I love about yoga and Yoga Nidra is the idea that these practices don't give you anything you don't have already. Rather, they help you remove the layers that conceal your fundamental wholeness, a wholeness that has always been and will always be. Experiencing this wholeness boils down to Awareness, and Yoga Nidra is a very relaxing yet powerful way to develop your Awareness.

Chapter 24.
Stages Of Yoga Nidra

In yoga nidra we start with the outer grossest levels of our being, and gradually work our way inward.

The Eight Stages of Yoga Nidra

The eight stages of yoga nidra are meant to naturally lead your listeners to a hypnogogic state between sleep and normal wakefulness, where they can illumine the depths of the psyche and reveal any limiting beliefs, Self-defeating habits and tendencies, as well as have a direct experience of their own true inner nature.

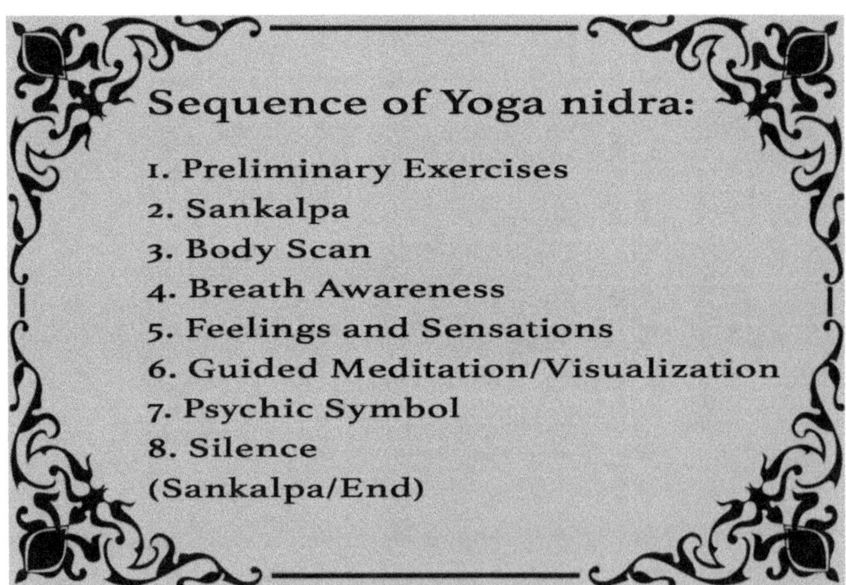

By becoming still and silent you are able to receive intuitions from your unconscious mind and find all the answers to your problems within your own Self. Others can always misguide you; even the most well-trained psychotherapists, but the inner revelations you receive from your highest Self will never lead you astray.

The eight stages of yoga nidra lead your participants deeper and deeper into their own selves where they can encounter their own true nature as totally liberated and perfectly blissful Spirit, thus empowering them to live more meaningful lives in whatever current circumstances they may find themselves in.

The inner peace experienced during yoga nidra transfer over into every other area of our lives, psychologically, emotionally and even for our physical health by eliminating all tension and stress. We subconsciously clench and hold stress in the neuromuscular system of our physical body; yoga nidra begins the process of unwinding and relearning how to release habitual nervous tension and stress.

Your participants come into a state of perfect relaxation combined with total awareness, which allows them to transcend the gross conscious state of mind and explore the subconscious and unconscious dimensions while fully awake.

Ultimately, the purpose behind yoga nidra is to structure the opportunity for your listeners to have their own personal experience. This inner experience is more likely to happen in the silent spaces between each instruction, and each instruction should be spoken in a way to lead your listeners to the next phase of silence where they can have the experiences you are describing for themselves.

For this reason, the silence between instructions is just as important as the words you speak.

Preparatory Exercises

A full yoga nida session is typically between twenty and forty minutes, however, there really is no limit. The duration will depend on the setting, context and ability of your participants.

The very first stage of yoga nidra is the preparation exercises. Here you ask your participants to lie down in shavasana, corpse pose, and assume a symmetrical position by spreading their arms and legs a comfortable distance apart. You tell them to adjust and become comfortable one last time before beginning the practice.

The purpose for the preparation exercises are to lead your listeners to become as comfortable as possible, while interrupting the habitual thought patterns so that they are more able to listen to your instructions. One way of interrupting the habitual thought patterns of your listeners is to instruct them to listen to any various sounds in their environment, ask them to perceive any sound or silence they may perceive outside the building you are in, inside the building and, in advanced stages, within their own bodies.

You ask your listeners to focus on the raw qualities of sounds without any past associations attached to them because this requires them to listen so intently that they must silence all other thoughts to the exclusion of whatever sound they happen to be perceiving.

Encourage them to listen to these sounds as if they have never heard them before, as if they were totally foreign and new. This can be a fun game to play with yourself and makes it easier to listen to the quality of sounds we typically attribute as being mundane, such as the sound of a fan or air conditioner, or the sound of traffic outside.

All sounds are only energy, and energy is neutral; it is the mind that makes it pleasant or unpleasant, good or bad.

After some time of listening to external sounds, the mind becomes disinterested in the outer world and is now ready to withdraw the senses and really begin the process of relaxing and listening to your instructions.

Beginning the Actual Practice

The next stage of yoga nidra, stage two, is when yoga nidra truly begins. Now that your listeners are relaxed both physically and mentally, you can plant the seed of sankalpa. A sankalpa is your determined resolve to achieve something, become something or experience something great. It is more than a desire or intention. It is your firm determined willpower concentrated into a single potent statement. When you know what you want in life without any doubt, and you are working towards that with all your energy and focus every day, the words to your sankalpa will come to you spontaneously. Until then, it is better to choose a positive affirmation.

You may want to consider facilitating an entire yoga nidra session only devoted towards helping your participants discover their own sankalpa.

After the sankalpa, the nest stage is body scan, where you will begin rotating the awareness around the various body parts, always in a set definite pattern. Do not change the pattern that you do body scan. Traditionally we start at the right-hand thumb and hit all the major body parts along the right side of the body, terminating at the right small toe. Then the next circuit begins at the left-hand thumb and progresses in the same pattern to the left small toe. Subsequent circuits proceed from the top of the head, down the facial features, all the way down the front side of the torso to the legs and toes. There is also the backside of the body, the organs and the major groupings of body parts altogether. (Refer to the scripts in the appendixes for a complete description of the body scan technique).

Traditionally the rotation of awareness around the body is done rapidly, however, I have found that a lot of people get anxious when you move at a fast speed, so in my own yoga nidra sessions I have added three to four seconds of silence between each body part to make it more calming and soothing. However, that adds a lot of time to the yoga nidra session, and it will be difficult to end a full session in less than forty-five minutes.

If you want to have shorter sessions you will need to oscillate the awareness around the body at a faster rate, in which case, you can give your listeners a fair warning by saying something such as: 'During body scan you will be asked to rotate your awareness around the body from part to part very quickly and rapidly, do not allow your awareness to spend too much time at one body part, but feel the momentum of energy flowing swiftly with the awareness from body part to body part, starting with... the right hand thumb' and continue.

Next, in stage four we begin breath awareness. At this point the body has effectively been put to sleep and we are working on bringing stillness and tranquility to the energy body, characterized by the breath and emotions. The breath and the emotions are intimately tied to each other, as one goes - so goes the other. In yoga nidra we do not do conscious breathing, we merely become aware of the spontaneous rhythms of each breath; like a surfer riding on the wave of the breath, not trying to change it, or alter it, merely flowing along with it united as one.

In stage six of yoga nidra you introduce a series of visualizations to your listeners. The items you ask them to visualize often have a universal archetypal significance and are meant to stir and awaken the deeper centers of the psyche. Images you will ask your participants to visualize include landscapes, famous monuments such as the pyramids, oceans, mountains, deserts, ancient monolithic temples at dawn, saints and flowers, stories from the Upanishads or Puranas, and powerful descriptions of psychic symbols such as Aum, or psychic centers such as the chakras and nadis.

The purpose for the visualization stage is to relax the mind fully. The visualizations lead the mind deeper within, where it can become relaxed and single-pointed. This single pointedness is the stage of dharana that naturally leads to meditative states and eventually, Samadhi.

In stage seven, you introduce the final visualization. The final visualization is given as a support for meditation. It is the base of concentration the mind focuses on while becoming more one-pointed and serene. The mind needs an object to focus on, so the final visualization should be something that is pleasant and powerful, such as a vision of an endless vast dark blue Ocean under a cloudy night sky, with rolling waves, rolling on and on endlessly across the surface of the sea.

Finally, you will begin to call your listeners back to this world, this present time and location. Lead them to repeat their sankalpa one more time; this is the perfect time to reap the fruits of sankalpa. Next you guide them to visualize the room they are lying in, and their own body lying on the floor. Tell them to keep their eyes shut and only move one single finger at first. Then another, and finally, to wiggle their fingers and toes, stretch and open their eyes to end the session.

As is traditional, I end all my sessions with a blessing for peace by saying the Sanskrit word for peace, shanti, three times with meaning.

Chapter 25.
The Art Of Relaxation

Inducing Yoga Nidra, or full body relaxation, becomes easy with practice. It's a skill that you must learn if you want to maximize your hidden potentials. It may be difficult at first, but the benefits are tremendous and promising. You can do Yoga Nidra alone, but the best way for beginners is to have a Yoga Nidra teacher who can guide you properly. Should you decide to do it alone, here are some steps that you should follow:

Step #1 – Lie down or sit down comfortably

Lie down comfortably in a supine position (lying down on your back, face up). Use a soft pillow to support your head. You can also use another one to support your knees. Another alternative is to sit on a chair with a back rest. Your back should be supported comfortably. Use a blanket to cover your body if it's cold.

Step #2 – Do some stretches

Perform some basic stretches to help loosen the body. You can do some arm and leg stretches, mentally preparing yourself to relax. For arm stretches, you can stretch your arm over your head several times or stretch them sideways or forward. You can do that similarly with your legs. You need not go into heavy aerobic exercises or strenuous sports for this step.

Step #3 – Focus on your selected object of relaxation

Teachers use different methods to induce relaxation, and they'll guide you through their particular process. But since you're doing it alone, choose a sound that can work well with you. You can play soft music, listen to a ringing bell, or listen to sound waves, whichever is most effective for you. You may opt to hear your voice reciting one or two words repeatedly.

Step #4 – Start focusing on the parts of your head

Close your eyes and focus on the various parts of your head, from the top of your head to your chin. Observe the sensations in your mouth and tongue. Take note of the air passing in and out of your nostrils. Include your eyebrows, cheekbones and forehead in your observations. What are the sensations you're feeling? Observe yourself as a third party would. Be aware of all the feelings occurring in the different parts of your face.

Step #5 – Focus on your upper torso

Now, mentally go further down to your neck and then off to your fingertips. Focus on each of the parts in your upper torso such as your neck, shoulders, arms, elbows, hands, wrists, fingers and fingertips, all one by one. Feel each sensation in these body parts as an observer. You'll have to observe each of these body parts. Do this several times while inhaling and exhaling. Feel the air and blood going down to your fingertips and then up your hand, wrist, arm, shoulders and neck. Observe how your chest heaves up and down with each breath, imagining the air going through your body parts. End by focusing on your chest.

Step #6 – Focus on your lower torso

You now mentally move your focus down further into your lower torso. This includes your stomach, abdomen, lower back, thighs, knees, calves, ankles, feet, and toes. Go through the same procedure as the upper torso. Inhale and exhale as you focus on each body part. Imagine the air coursing through each part. As you inhale, think about bringing in pure energy and as you exhale, imagine your body getting rid of all negative energy traits such as anxieties, worries, problems and stress. Continue this process going back and forth for at least a minute until you feel relaxed. Go back to your chest and feel the air leaving and entering your body. Repeat this action until you feel relaxed.

Step #7 – Do it all over again

Focus on the parts of your head again and repeat the same process as step #4. However, this time, observe first your right body parts, followed by your left body parts. The spaces in between these body parts should also be observed. Concentrate on the tiniest detail of your body like the tip of your fingers. Do this while you continue inhaling and exhaling and imagining that new energy is coming in while negative energy is going out. Repeat step #5 and #6 but focus on all the body parts on your right side first before proceeding to the left body parts. Be consciously aware of all the observations.

By this time, your body must be in a calm state. Some may fall asleep at this stage. If you fall asleep when you do it for the first time, it's okay. Keep doing it until you can fully complete the exercise without falling asleep.

Step #8 – Perform the spinal breath

Now, you will begin to perform spinal breathing by inhaling and feeling the air passing from the top of your head to the base of your spinal cord. Then, exhale as if the air is passing from the base of your spinal cord to the top of your head. Use your inner visualization to imagine your breath as a stream of silver going up and down your spine. Perform this several times as you relax your body.

Step #9 – Enter your Yoga Nidra

Before you enter your Yoga Nidra, ensure that your body is completely relaxed. If not, you have to repeat steps #3 to #8, until you achieve total relaxation. When you're certain you're ready, you can now enter your Yoga Nidra. Some prefer to enter Yoga Nidra in silence. So, if you have a friend nearby, you can ask him to turn off any sound silently when you're about to enter Yoga Nidra. If this is not possible, then try to select relaxation prompts that do not distract you in any way, or ones that will turn themselves off after a certain period.

First, focus on the space between your eyebrows. Concentrate on this space for 5 to 10 minutes. Afterwards, move your focus down to your throat and concentrate on the center of your throat for several minutes, until you find that you can concentrate effortlessly. You can then proceed to focus on the space between your breasts and then to the center of your heart. Get rid of all thoughts, sensations and emotions. Let go of anything in your heart and mind and simply delve deeper into the silence of your inner self. Maintain this state for at least 10 minutes.

As you gain more experience practicing Yoga Nidra, you

can lengthen the time of stillness and silence. What's important is that you have truly achieved a total relaxation of mind, body and soul. Through this, you can train your subconscious to be in congruence with your conscious mind. In this way, you greatly increase your ability to fulfill your desires and life goals. This stems from the fact that the subconscious will also have the same goal as your conscious – meaning that your subconscious will find all possible ways and means to manifest itself outwardly.

Step #10 – Return to full consciousness

During your first-time practicing Yoga Nidra, you may have a shorter time span to get back to full consciousness. As soon as thoughts start coming into your mind, acknowledge them and slowly return to your consciousness. You can start this by opening your eyes, wiggling your toes or stretching your arms. There are no contraindications to Yoga Nidra but only health benefits because you're able to reduce your stress and anxiety levels. However, you should take note that various teachers tend to modify some steps depending on their experiences and preferences.

While performing the steps before Yoga Nidra, your focus may be interrupted with other thoughts, so you have to re-focus every time. This takes practice, so don't despair if you can't concentrate during the first time that you perform the exercises. Eventually, you'll come to develop a sharper inner eye and a more focused mind. When you experience a distracting thought, just nip it away as soon as you can, and move back to focusing on your body parts in the sequence described herein.

Chapter 26.
Training The Mind

Meditating is one of the ways which relaxes the mind and shuts out the whole world from it. You only get to focus on only one single thought, and in this case, you should be focusing on positive and beautiful thoughts, filling your mind with them. In meditating, you should be in a relaxed state of mind and in a calm environment away from the hustle and bustle of active life. If you live in the city or in a busy town, it is advisable that you find a calm, quiet and tranquil space from where you can meditate in. The sole purpose of meditating is clearing up the toxic thoughts and images in our heads, and this efficiently achieved when one is in a calm environment. Also, when doing your meditation, ensure that you have ample time with you; that you are not in a rush to work or engagement, so that it will not be in a hurried manner. This might not actually work, for it does not fulfill the purpose of meditating. You can also have your clothes as lose and fitting, to free your physical body as it aids in also freeing your mental state. When you are meditating, block out all the negative thoughts and energy and focus on staying on the positive border of thoughts. Do this consistently, and you'll be having positive and beautiful images in your mind, even when not meditating. On the aspect of yoga, the workouts are a great sport for relieving stress and the negativity from your brain through the physical exercises. Yoga increases the consciousness in an individual, translating you to a higher consciousness in nature. By cultivating such consciousness, positivity is enriched in the brain as you work out. As much as yoga is great for physical wellness, it is also equally nourishing to the brain, instilling positive vibes in an individual. Both yoga and meditation go hand in hand in uplifting your mental state, thus your thoughts being those of positive and beautiful things, helping your mind to focus, as they both demand great time spans of full concentration and attention from a person.

Smile often

Smiling often is a cure to negative thoughts, and a single smile can distill all the negativity you had. Smiling requires no effort, absolutely. You neither have to go to the gym nor do you have to be in a tranquil place, as in meditation to do so. Feeling low? Turn the frown into a smile. It's just moving the facial muscles, and you are okay again. Smiling has a way of making you happier and lighter and less burdened if you were feeling heavy burdened. Bearing happier results to more positivity in life; therefore, your goal of projecting positive and beautiful images in your mind is achieved. When you smile, you also become more productive, for positive emotions are playing out inside you. They fuel you to work harder and in a more efficient way, staying focused on a task for the required time without being distracted, thus being productive. That's how far a smile can go in changing the direction of your day and uplifting your mood if you were low. Having emotions bordering on the happy side makes you view things on the bright side of life, which streams from having a positive mindset within you. As stated, smiling does away with all the negative and the draining emotions in you, leaving you lighter. It does away with the pain you could be experiencing. When you have not positive images in your mind and feeling less focused, stand before a mirror and will yourself to smile. You will feel the energy shift immediately. You will feel more rejuvenated, more up to the task. Do not just will with your mind of a physical smile on your face for that will not be productive, will it spring forth from within, for from such it will positively impact your mind.

Have positive and focused likeminded people around you

By being surrounded by positive energy all around you from your friends and family, you will surely also have the same positive energy vibe. This will go a long way in projecting positive images to your brain in the long run, that produces positive energy. As a smile is contagious, so can positivity and negativity be. They are vibes that can be transferred to you without really knowing, but you will feel of the effects later. A company of negative minded people will transform you to be always seeing the negative side of things. Conversely, positive people have an impact on you to see the brighter side of life. They smile more, they laugh more and generally take life at a lighter note, which is needed to projector beautiful images in your mind. Surround yourself with such. Determined and strong-willed people are also another category that pushes you to be focused and be the best that you can be. Not being content with the status quo, they strive further to reach the highest attainable standards, without exerting and expending too much of their energy. Being in the company of likeminded people will give you the drive to be focused on whatever activity you undertake to achieve excellent results.

Change your negative thoughts to positive ones

Having a change in your negative thoughts to positive ones have a general effect on your outlook on situations and life in general. Positive thoughts reflect in the images that are projected to your mind. Negative thoughts tend to bring you down and can lead to a state of a near depression, for they just focus on the bad on everything. They do not give the good in life a chance. To have positive and beautiful thoughts, have an actual change from thinking to the negative side and start visualizing and living on the positive side. It is also true that negative minded people do not have the drive to work, the drive for life. With negativity clouding your mind, you will just be a dead man walking, having lost the drive to find your true purpose in life. Being focused cannot be achieved in such a state. You will be just telling yourself to be focused and determined and give your all in whatever you are working at, but you have no will to follow through the plan in your head. The lack of results due to your mindset may discourage you further and push you to fully abandon hope in dreaming and realizing your dreams in life. With a change to the positive mindset camp, things will seem simpler, even though, in reality, they are not. You will be facing the same challenges, but because of the change in attitude, you will come up with better ways to deal with them. More focus on your work will result from positivity.

Take charge of your own life

Be responsible for your own life and the activities that occur in your everyday life. Being responsible in this case means planning for your life, and not living just for the sake of living, but having a purpose of doing so. The accomplishment of your life goals will bring a sense of satisfaction to you. Being satisfied and feeling accomplished will project positivity in your mind and encourage you to be more focused. Start on this by having a journal and a planner. The journal is for entering the daily events of your day, how it rolled out, and whether you were successful in doing what you had planned to accomplish for the day. You write how the activities ensued, your positive and negative moments, and whether generally, the day was a win for you. It is to be done at the close of the day when you are retiring for the night. A journal entry will help you show how you can increase your positivity and in the accomplishment of your goals by staying more focused. A planner, on the other hand, is for you to write down all that you intend to do and achieve for that specific day. You can also set annual, monthly, and weekly goals that you intend to meet. This is one of the ways that you can take charge of your life. Plan meticulously, engaging your mind in every step of the way, and promising yourself that you are going to get the activities done. In this way, you push yourself to be focused on meeting your set goals. By analyzing your planner, you can see the activities you did and did not do. There is a feeling of happiness and giddiness that one gets when you have accomplished whatever you set out to do for the day. Beautiful projections are therefore made in your mind. Stay positive in this manner, planning and encouraging yourself daily. Taking charge of your life also means not letting bad situations bring you down. As earlier mentioned, fill your mind with positive thoughts. When the wave of negativity threatens to crash, take charge of your life by being focused on having positive images in your mind.

Singing

Singing can be classified into one category as smiling. It has instant relief over a weary soul when the right kind of music is put on. Even when you are not down or low, good music totally applies to project positive and beautiful images in mind. From the lyrics of the song, the mind forms images of whatever scenario is playing out in the song. When a good-spirited song is on, good images will form in the mind of the listener. Not only do you have to listen to music, sing along with it. This is the essence of good lyrics intended to make you better. It is also not necessary for you to sing along with music that you have blasted on, you can also sing from your memory. Singing out aloud is the best way of instilling positive images in mind. Most often than not, you can always relate to whatever the singer has written and more or less had the same experience. With a happy song, you will tend to reminisce of the happy times that you have had, putting a smile on your face in the process and creating beautiful images in your mind. Songs are surely a great tool that moves our minds. Even with the uplifting that good songs have on you, you have to be wary of songs that are depressing and draining. Such kind of songs tends to bring down a person, with their beats and their depressing words. When choosing to sing a song or play music, do choose one with positive vibes. Some people are also unique in such a way that they cannot perform any task without music or singing or humming a tune. If you are one of those people, have music play when you work, inspiring music, to keep you focused and increase your attention on your work.

Be an avid reader of positive quotes

Positive quotes are one of the most favorite places for

people to stop by and feel re-inspired and rejuvenated. There are quotes about everything, and since you are seeking positive and beautiful images in your mind, focus on the ones that offer positivity and focused content. There are lots of them on the internet, and in print form, quotes have been published. You can, therefore, have access to many quotes at the tip of your hands. Many writers have invested in writing quotes that buoy your spirits up, and that feels me good, and you are instantly feeling better, in a better and lighter mood, feeling at the top of the world, like you can conquer anything. Well, those are really good at motivating you to give your best in everything you do, making you stay focused on your activities and feel accomplished at the end of the day. The most common quotes on the internet and the in books are happy quotes. Read them to form beautiful images in your mind. Many of these quotes are always done in a poetic manner that make them appealing to read. They should, therefore, not be boring to go over. You can have a site that you can subscribe to, to be getting daily quotes on happiness and positivity, and staying focused on your work. Most of these sites writing on quotes on the internet are mostly free, and the subscription is only via email or by getting an app. It's pretty an easy way of having happiness and positive lines being given to you every morning when you wake. It sets out your day for a positive mentality. You can also have the settings to make the notifications in a span of several hours in a day, such that in a single day, you will get several quotes to keep you going until the day ends. You need beautiful images in your mind, read quotes on beautiful things, and the images will be translated. Need a dose of positivity in your life, read quotes on staying positive. Simply, in the area that you lack energy in, get yourself a quote to keep you going.

Be grateful

Being grateful is an attribute that improves your outlook in life and prevents you from wallowing in self-pity over whatnots in your life. Being grateful as an individual is acknowledging whatever you have and appreciating its value, from material possessions such as an apartment, a car, to immaterial ones such as friendships, bonds, and family. Being grateful is a choice that you make not to look at the negativities that are going in your life but rather on the good that you already have and being content with it. This does not mean that you are not to deal with problems and challenges because of the reason; being grateful. It, however, means that you acknowledge that there is a challenge, yes, but you choose not to dwell on it too much, letting it suck up your positive energy and drain you emotionally. Instead, it's choosing to focus more on what you've got right now, than whatever you don't have, or you have lost. Gratitude for things will make you realize how privileged you are and not take things for granted. Coming to the realization of how blessed you are, you will be oozing of positivity. Your mind will be transformed to have a positive outlook on everything, appreciating even the small, minute random things that are done to us or that we have. Being content in your soul over what you have and not being troubled over your challenge's washes over a certain kind of peace in you. Beautiful, kind, and good things will have filled your mind, with no room of negative and sad thoughts. Always take a moment or two to think about the situations that other people go through so that you realize you are not badly off, then you can also sing it off, as a crowning feature of the positivity inside your soul.

Move on after a negative setback

We are all prone to failure, to setbacks, to disappointments. But what is of great importance is the way in which we deal with that kind of heart-wrenching drawbacks and how we move on with our lives, whether a file with negativity or a change to the positive outlook in life. To get positive images in your mind, you have to pick up yourself from the failure you had encountered, dust yourself, as a common quote says, and go on living positively. How you deal with setbacks is the determinant of what your mind projects in you. How you move on after a drawback also determines the kind of output, you'll be having in your work area. Letting the experience scar you to the point of negligence on yourself stems from a place of negativity. Concentrate on building up yourself again with positive thoughts and vibe as the building blocks. As mentioned earlier, read positive, happy, feel-good quotes, play, and sing along to songs that are uplifting, meditate, do yoga, and other activities to get you back on the track. The mind is a result of what you feed it. Feed it beautiful and positive things, and you'll get the same output being reflected by it.

Be kind and helpful

This is one of the aspects of projecting positive and beautiful things in our minds and staying focused that does not deal with yourself only. By making others grow, by helping others, you, in turn, get to be surrounded by positivity and the same in your mind. You can find activities that you can do to help someone. It may not always be a far-fetched idea as feeding the hungry and the poor but also minute actions of kindness in our everyday lives. Well, feeding the poor and sheltering the homeless is also another great way of helping people who are in need. By giving out a piece of kindness from our hearts to those in need of it, prompts the mind to project love, kindness, and goodness. You will also feel good about yourself about doing these little acts of love and kindness to people who deserve them. You can also go further and offer them hugs as a sign of affection to them. Charity, the greatest form of humanity that the world is need of at the current world, will have been offered to a broken human being, whom you'll have started healing by that simple act. More positivity from you to the world and more positivity from within you. Beautiful images will always be in your mind as a result of your actions.

Chapter 27.
Pratyahara

Pratyahara (withdrawal of the senses), dharana (concentration) and dhyana (meditation) make up the fifth, sixth and seventh limbs of Patanjali's astanga marga, Eight-Limbed Raja Yoga path. The three limbs of pratyhara, dharana and dhyana, when practiced correctly, is a seamless transition. Pratyhara naturally leads to dharana, and dharana naturally leads to dhyana. When this is accomplished, it will naturally lead to the state of Samadhi, the eighth limb. We will explore these sadhanas below.

After we are steady in asana and are aligned with the Cosmos, we practice pranayama to purify the nadis so we can guide energy through them. By observing the flow of prana, we come to understand how it moves throughout the body, both nourishing it and also clearing energy obstructions in the nadis. Once we are established thus, in pranayama, it is advised to pursue the sadhana of pratyahara, dharana and dhyana. These sadhanas are part of the natural progression in the path of yoga and may initially seem obscure, but they will become clearer as you advance in your yoga practice.

Pratyahara

In Sanskrit, pratyahara generally refers to withdrawal of the senses and is associated with prana shakti and chit shakti, described below. As per the astanga marga of Maharishi Patanjali, he describes pratyahara as a bridge between bahiranga (external) aspects of yoga and the antharanga (internal) yoga. With pratyahara we are moving our consciousness to an internal state away from the external senses. Each of our five external senses (sight, sound, taste, smell, and touch) provide our consciousness with information regarding the external physical world, and they are powered by prana shakti (the power or directing/driving force behind prana) when it is outwardly focused. Pratyahara is the process of recalling the outwardly dispersed prana shakti to return to its abode in the heart to allow us to change our focus to the internal world, which we are often not in tune with. Due to externalization of the senses, we become distracted from our true nature and become lost in the world of duality. By drawing the prana shakti back to the heart, we can dispel the ignorance (the perception of duality) and understand our true nature.

Patanjali describes prathyahara as the natural occurrence after fruitful practice of pranayama; however, there are other methods, in addition to pranayama, which have been developed for the practice of prathyahara.

Though in many books it is mentioned that there are six major chakras in the human being, viz. muladhara, swadhisthana, manipura, anahata, visuddha and ajna before reaching the sahasrara, there are many chakras (points of nadi junctions) all over the body. Through visualization and consistent practice, one can draw the prana, by the aid of chit shakti (power or directing/driving force of consciousness or will), step by step to the chosen point of concentration. When this is accomplished, the senses and sense perceptions are gradually severed from the mind, resulting in a calm and serene mental state. The chit shakti is the tool we use to guide the prana shakti according to our will.   We use the practice of dharana to hone this tool to its maximum potential.

Dharana

Directing our consciousness to a place without distraction is dharana. In simple words, dharana is concentration of our chit shakti in one place without distraction of sense perceptions.

Where is this place?   It can be anywhere, within or outside our body. In pratyahara, we have drawn our consciousness back to the root by directing our sense perceptions inward. The five senses that distract our consciousness and do not allow us to look inward and concentrate are drawn-back.

Where can we concentrate? We can concentrate on inner light by directing our vision in any place in the body, like between the eyebrows or at the center of the heart. Otherwise we can concentrate on external objects like a flower, a small spot on the wall, the moon, or the stars (especially a small blinking star).   We can also concentrate on inner sound, by focusing first on the subtle, then subtler and finally the subtlest sounds of our inner self. Or we can concentrate on our breath or a mantra we utter inwardly.

In other words, the concentration unifies the five sense limbs, five sense perceptions, the mind, the intellect, the will and the ego. To attune your chit shakti you have to practice dharana in the ways mentioned above. Once it is attuned it is easier to draw the prana shakti to a chosen point of concentration.

Dhyana

When we achieve dharana (concentration in one point as explained above), and strive to prolong the concentration, it will result in merging the observer and the observed. In this state duality vanishes into non-duality. This prolonged state of concentration is dhyana, the seventh limb, which brings the chit-shakti and prana shakti together. In this way we can achieve the state of dhyana, which is otherwise known as meditation.

A mere state of temporary calmness, dreaminess or other similar states are often incorrectly defined as meditation. Only the state of dhyana mentioned above can be called meditation in its true sense.

How does one practice prathyahara, dharana and dhyana as a seamless transition? After fruitful practice of pranayama, sit in any meditative asana such as siddhasana, swastikasana or sukhasana. Use the chit shakti as a tool to draw the prana shakti through the nadis. Select either anahata chakra (heart area) or ajna chakra (slightly above and between the eyebrows), or sahasrara (top of head) as your point of concentration. Feel and visualize the entire body pulsating with prana shakti. Now we will begin to pull the prana shakti from the toes of the feet and fingers of the hands to our chosen point of concentration.

First slowly draw back the prana shakti from the toes to the calves and from the fingers to the forearms. Next draw it from the calves to the knees and from the forearms to the elbows. Slowly and steadily keep drawing it step by step closer to the point of concentration.

Along with the prana shakti we will be withdrawing our sense perceptions inward to the point of concentration. Once the prana shakti of our entire body reaches our point of concentration, we are closed to the external world and have internalized our consciousness. Prolong the concentration and try to see whatever is visible internally, hear whatever is audible internally and feel any internal sensations. Initially, we may be able to concentrate only for a few seconds without distraction, but through regular practice we are able to hold the concentration steady for several minutes. At that stage, the observer and the observed merge and become one.

For achieving the state of dhyana, we should be firmly established in asana and all our nadis should be cleansed by the practice of pranayama. This is why pranayama is so important, and why purification is critical to the success of yoga. Without enough purification, the nadis are blocked and prana shakti cannot be drawn through them.

A Special Note About Samadhi

Samadhi is referred to as the eighth limb and is the natural fruit of successful yoga, if the preceding seven limbs have been achieved with proficiency. There is no one single practice or training for the state of Samadhi. It is a spontaneous state beyond our limited 4-dimensional range of perception of mind and intellect. In this state, one's individual ego merges with Universal Ego; the observer, the observed and the process of observation cease to exist. It can also be thought of as union with God or becoming one with God. Words fail to express this state. The only indication of achieving this state is the bliss one experiences.

Chapter 28.
Yoga Sutras

The founder of the sutras string of knowledge is Maharishi Patanjali, who is equally regarded as the father of yoga. In as much as very little is known about Patanjali, many people are of the belief that he is thought to have existed somewhere in between 200 to 500 B.C. An era when the Ayurveda was the best form of wisdom that people had as the cure or remedy for their illnesses. Maharishi Patanjali brought forth this high-powered knowledge which later came to acquire the name Yoga Sutras.

During those contemporary days, virtually all the teachings were administered orally, and students learned through a process referred to as sutra. Sutra is a word that originates from the same "pot" as the term suture which is usually used in the medical field. It means holding together or creating a connection. Whenever a tutor expounded on a given piece of information, the learners would be presented with a brief phrase that would, later, remind them of the greater material body. This was somewhat similar to the cue cards in the modern world. However, the problem is that in as much as somebody can have knowledge of the sutras, he/she can never comprehend or be certain of its greater understanding.

This probably explains the origin of the goat yoga in the modern-day.

Sankhya is part of the contemporary systems of philosophy in India. Theoretically, it has an understanding that knowledge is the gateway to enlightenment. Maharishi Patanjali's amazing gift to the universe was that he made use of this deep-rooted— and yet completely intelligent philosophy and converted or simplified it in a way that normal spiritual seeker could use and follow. A blueprint for your path to eventual enlightenment.

Taking into consideration that falling sick is not just the illness in the body, but is equally a representation of the ailments in the emotions and mind, the yoga sutras of Patanjali brings forth knowledge that does not merely administer cure to the body but also works on purifying the emotions, the mind as well as the entire existence itself, by using yoga.

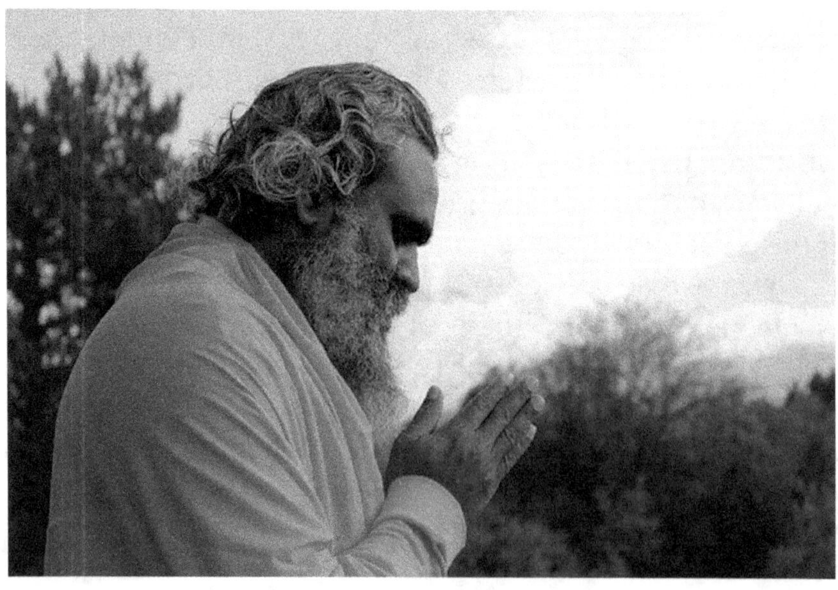

The Yoga Sutras

The aims of practicing yoga, how yogic powers develop and lastly, liberation. Just like a tender guiding stick, the yoga sutras caution you of the pitfalls on the spiritual voyage and consequently give you the strategies or ways in which you can vanquish or overpower them.

What Is the Essentiality of Your Spiritual Practices?

Your spiritual activities should aim at looking at your inner self. The real version of yourself is hidden in the tranquility of your thoughts, beyond all obstructions. Nonetheless, the confusion, chaos, and doubts within your thoughts push you to forget your true self.

The main hindrance to spiritual advancement is stress. It causes fatigue, resulting in laziness and doubts which push you to lose the meaning of who you really are. Staying committed to your practices is the perfect recipe to win this battle.

If you wish to achieve peace of mind, you should put into practice friendly attitudes without envying the people who are truly happy. Be merciful to the less fortunate and unhappy people, cherish show support to acts of virtuousness and practice impartiality to get rid of the dramas that the impure brings forth.

The outcome of the wrong action is misery and the outcome of virtuous actions is a joy. You must be responsible for words, actions, and thoughts by choosing to live consciously. The yoga sutras are the gateway to refinement, surrender, and purification.

Yoga Is Not the Condition of Being Alienated Spiritually

Patanjali gives a description of the flickering operations of these mind field fractures by naming them according to their category and type. In this part, we will bear witness to the controversy that has cropped up between the radical revolutionary academic reductionist school of dualism that follows the first narration or explanation of the Yoga Sutras (Vyasa) elucidation in contradiction to the real words of Patanjali. This is evident all through the sutras. It is the comprehension of these translators that the Yoga Sutra of Patanjali is not a book that talks about philosophy and that instead, it is intended to be entirely a guide book similar to the spirit of the manual of a lab to aid and accompany experimental practices. Therefore, for the novices, this is the toughest part of the whole Yoga Sutras if we chose to do a correlative study.

To clarify verses 1.5 to 11 of the Yoga Sutras, Patanjali is giving an address about the citta-vrtti (how our minds tend to dart from one thought to another) as well as how to unshackle our minds from their curtailment. He does not state anywhere that the vrtti are only five, but he categorically says that they can be classified or arranged in a manner that involves positioning them into five feasible categories. The majority of the vrtti are in existence as permutations or combinations of two or probably more of these fundamental categories and therefore the classical papers affirm that the count of vrtti is at 84,000.

This point is compelling for the simple fact that vrtti (though patterns that have been conditioned) can assume various forms. Most of us have had an experience of vrtti, virtually all the time, only excluding the infrequent moments of vision, inspiration, clarity, revelation, beauty, or meditation. However, the repressive problem usually takes place because when citta-vrtti is in a state of dominance, we are usually not aware of its operation and us also not aware of its coloring consequences; that is, we do not have the ability to go outside or beyond it to take note of its effects. Therefore, somebody who is mindful or somebody who meditates begins to take note of the rise and fall of the vrtta. There is no need for focusing om or following the vrtti, instead, you should realize that one is working or operating and make a choice to let it go. Do not give it attention. In the long run, through constant awareness, the vrtta do not have the power to mislead or occlude the midfield. An individual becomes used to in the real nature of his/her own mind which is basically the truthful nature of every prevalent all-mind.

Therefore, vrtti does not designate some theoretical concept of intellectuality, instead it gives a description of our thought design that possess or occupies our minefields of being attentive- any restricting procedure of patterning that obscures, colors, limits, perverts, corrupts prejudices, restricts, or restrains our experience of our intrinsic truthful nature, infinite mind, or original mind as well as the greatest potential to solve. The main reason why recognizing vrtta is essential because vrtti brings forth emotional and mental afflictions. Both are initially recognized in an orderly manner to get rid of them, however, they are not accorded any focus. Slowly, they undergo attenuation and then they are entirely set free in functional yoga.

Yoga Practices Starting with the Most Important

Patanjali categorically states that the essence behind yoga practices are the vigorous focused on commitment to results. Therefore, yoga is a practice that is process-oriented and not a practice that is goal-oriented. If practicing yoga is deeply rooted in original liveliness that is non-dual, then the view is in the path and in turn, the path shows the fruit. It is not focused on achieving a certain goal, but it simply permits the deepening of innate, non-dual and natural compassion and luminosity to shine, as the fraudulent identifications and barriers are set free. Simply put, in times of process orientation, the fruit is usually in plain sight as it offers guidance to the practice. The conditions are often boundless.

The intensification levels of not being attached to events and objects are revealed and clarified until the highest level of freedom of release is achieved. This is finished with the remarkable surrender of the mindset of egoism and selfish motivation.

Failing this deliverance through remarkable non-attachment to certain objects, then Patanjali insists that somebody should intensify his/her practice. Later, in the book, we will see that yoga sutra fundamentally deals with cutting lose our fetishes and attachments on objects; hard or even extremely soft. This manner of surrendering to the highest of personal luminous love can be used in almost all yogic practices

Putting Patanjali's Yoga Sutra into Practice

In the Yoga Sutra, Patanjali says that if we wish to achieve a powerful foundation, we have to practice for long periods of time without being interrupted, having belief in it as well as anticipating it with the mindset of service. The first ground rule that Patanjali offers is a long time (Digha-Kala). This means that taking note of what you are undertaking is not something that can be achieved overnight. You have to be committed for a long time to get almost permanent results that you will be proud of.

Therefore, any time you do something g new, irrespective of whether it is a job or a relationship, Patanjali advises you to be ready to put in some effort.

Chapter 29.
A Different Kind Of Yoga

Like life, yoga is an ongoing quest to find balance. Compared with other forms of yoga and physical activity that strengthen muscles, yin yoga stretches and stimulates what's deeper beneath the surface: the connective tissues in the body. Yin is a slower-paced practice, with an emphasis on spending a long time in postures and cultivating stillness.

Practicing with Yin and Yang

The wisdom of ancient Chinese philosophy states that all things in the universe have opposing energies: yin and yang. The common symbol taijitu illustrates this concept with a black-and-white circle with a spiral pattern inside, representing how these contrasting energies are always intertwined and flowing into each other. The yang, or white side of the symbol, often represents brightness, masculinity, rigidity, and mobility, while the yin, or black side, represents darkness, femininity, softness, and immobility. In applying this context to the physical body, our muscles are considered yang, and the connective tissues that make up our tendons, ligaments, and bones are considered yin.

Our muscles respond well to dynamic, repetitive movements. Think about your last visit to the gym. Though you may have been exhausted after your workout with weights or your run on the treadmill, your muscles were able to withstand the activity. In fact, a big reason why you continue to work out may be because you can see the benefits it has on your body as your muscles grow bigger and become stronger.

On the other hand, the connective tissues do not respond well to being stressed in the same active, repetitive manner. But all too often we engage the entire body in high-intensity, dynamic movements while neglecting to explore the benefits of gentler, passive stretching. This is where yin yoga comes in.

Yin yoga draws on the concepts that yin and yang energies form a whole and that the interaction and coexistence of the opposites are essential to creating a mind and body in balance. It is a highly beneficial practice of long-held passive stretches that intentionally target the deep connective tissues in the body that other dynamic forms of yoga and exercise do not reach.

THE BENEFITS OF YIN YOGA

Teaches the mind and body to be still: The long holds and contemplative nature of yin yoga are great training for a meditation practice. With stillness and surrender as objectives, you will learn to quiet the chatter in your mind and focus on the sensations in your body while remaining calm.

Reduces stress and anxiety: As a slower practice, yin activates the parasympathetic nervous system—also known as the body's rest and digest response—which lowers your heart rate, increases circulation, and stabilizes breathing for a more relaxed demeanor.

Strengthens connective tissue and joints: While a more active yoga practice targets the movement and contraction of our muscles (yang), the yin practice gently exercises our joints and surrounding connective tissues. Through the practice of holding postures for a longer time, yin yoga strengthens the connective tissue and increases the flexibility of the joints.

Improves mobility: Yin yoga postures primarily target the hips, low back, and pelvic areas—all areas that become less mobile with age. The gentle stretches of yin yoga help loosen fascia to bring more mobility around the muscles and ligaments in the body.

Promotes healthier organ function: Yin yoga fosters a still body and mindful breath, which enables blood to circulate more easily. Increased circulation nourishes and stimulates the organs.

What's Yoga Got to Do with Taoism?

It's no secret that yoga's origins are in India, so it may seem odd that yin yoga is heavily influenced by the Chinese philosophy of Taoism. But, in fact, Taoism and yoga share very similar principles.

Hatha is the type of yoga that is meant to calm your thoughts and align the mind and body (as opposed to vinyasa, which has a faster pace and is designed to build heat and strengthen muscles). In the word "hatha," ha refers to the energy of the sun while the reflects the energy of the moon. Furthermore, the root of the word "yoga" is yuj, which means "yoke" or "union." Like the

Taoist theory of yin and yang, the practice of hatha yoga is based on the union of the opposing energies of the sun and moon to bring balance. Therefore, the integration of yin and yang with hatha yoga is spot-on.

The yin yoga shared in this book is based on concepts explored and developed by several master teachers, including Paul Grilley (influenced by Paulie Zink and Dr. Hiroshi Motoyama), Bernie Clark, and Sarah Powers. They fuse elements of Taoism, traditional Chinese medicine, anatomy, and hatha yoga to create a style of yin yoga that is therapeutic, stimulating, and strengthening for the body.

QI THEORY

In yin yoga, poses are held in stillness for a long time in order to stimulate and stretch the deeper connective tissues. This action of holding postures helps move energy through the body. This energy is known as qi (or chi) in the tradition of Chinese medicine and as prana (or "life force") in the Indian yogic and Ayurvedic traditions, and it moves along a set of pathways in the body called meridians.

There are 12 main meridians that form a network connecting to the body's major organs. Yin yoga postures stretch the connective tissue along these meridian lines. As a result, the organs they serve are revitalized and rejuvenated by the flow of qi, leading to improved well-being in body, mind, and spirit.

Poses (Asanas)

Yin yoga poses generally aren't so different from the poses practiced in other forms of yoga, but there are a few special considerations to keep in mind.

Yin postures are generally done seated, while other yoga styles like Power Vinyasa or Bikram involve many standing sequences. Since yin poses often focus on the lower body (mainly the low back, hips, and legs), it's easier to hold the poses for an extended period while seated.

The alignment of a pose should not cause stress or pain to any area of the body. For example, if the intention of the pose is to stress the connective tissues of the hip joint, and the manner in which you take the pose causes pain in the knee area, you should modify the pose based on your personal anatomy to alleviate any pain.

In order to stress the deep connective tissues around a joint, you must keep those muscles relaxed while you hold a pose. If the muscles are tense, then the stretch won't target the connective tissues. It's important to note that the only muscles you need to relax while in a yin pose are the muscles specific to the focus area. For instance, if the pose focuses on the hips, it's not necessary to engage your arm muscles.

Yin poses involve long hold times. Once you've come into a pose and have arrived at your edge, it's time to become still and settle into the pose. You want to hold each pose for a challenging amount of time; you can hold them for as long as 20 minutes if you'd like. The long hold time not only allows the deep connective tissues (fascia, ligament, and bone) to be stressed and stretched to build deep inner strength but also promotes the therapeutic clearing of injuries, traumas, and repetitive movement patterns (such as sitting a certain way in a chair or always carrying a bag over the same shoulder) stored in the body.

In some cases, holding a yin pose can cause energy (qi) or blood to be restricted in certain areas. A yang pose is then provided as a follow-up to help get things moving again before the next long yin pose.

JOINT, TISSUE, AND LIGAMENT HEALTH

The idea of holding a yoga posture for a long time in order to stretch deep connective tissues may sound intimidating (or even unsafe) at first, but the truth is that yin yoga can improve the health of your joints, ligaments, and bones.

While we hold the posture in stillness, the deep stretching occurs from the stress, or tension, placed on the tissues. Although the most popular styles of exercise are yang-like and train the muscles through quick repetitive movements, yin yoga is often called the "quiet practice" because the results don't happen right away. However, over time the deeper connective tissues do become thicker, longer, and stronger.

Why is this beneficial to our health? As we age, we lose stability and mobility in our joints, and our bodies become stiffer. Cultivating stronger and elongated tissues through yin yoga helps us with mobility and flexibility as we age.

The Breath

As with other styles of yoga, breathing is a vital part of yin practice. The purpose of the breathing is to elicit calm and relaxation and to activate the parasympathetic nervous system, which signals to the body that you are okay and not in danger.

When you are in a stressful situation, the sympathetic

nervous system (or the body's fight, flight, or freeze response) automatically kicks in because your body is concerned about keeping you safe. When this system is activated, stress hormones are released, your heart rate increases, your muscles become tense, your blood pressure rises, and your breathing becomes rapid. This is the opposite of what you want to experience when practicing yin yoga. The parasympathetic nervous system, on the other hand, allows us to be calm and present in body and mind.

A yogic breathing style that is tremendously helpful for relaxation and calmness is the Ujjayi breath. Translated as "victorious breath," and often called the Ocean Breath, the Ujjayi technique involves guttural breathing during which you contract the glottis in the back of the throat to produce a soft, hissing sound for the exhalation. In more rigorous yang-like yoga practices, the expelling of the breath in Ujjayi can be harsh or loud. In yin, the objective is to keep the breath soft, rhythmic, and quiet. If that is not achievable for you with Ujjayi breathing, you can always use a calm, quiet breath with long inhalations and exhalations instead.

Though they are often linked together, yin yoga is not the same as restorative yoga. The intent of restorative yoga is full relaxation and surrender. To the contrary, the nature of the yin practice is stillness and presence. In yin practice, you are tuning in instead of tuning out.

WHEN TIME SLOWS DOWN

Yin poses are typically held for 3 to 5 minutes, but you can hold them for as long as 20 minutes.

Your experience of time in a pose can vary from day to

day depending on how you are feeling physically or emotionally. If you find it hard to stay in a pose once you've found your edge, it's best to come out of it. Stillness—not pain—is what's required.

Try setting a timer so you can stay focused in the practice. If your timer goes off and you want to hold the pose longer, go for it. Just be mindful of not overdoing it. Some signs that may indicate you have pushed your body too far are physical pain, spasms, tightness, or feeling out of alignment. If these appear, try backing off in the poses. Instead of taking a full expression of the pose, try a more moderate version and decrease the hold time. Gradually work your way back to longer holds. If it's altogether too difficult to practice at all, take care of yourself and give your body a break from practice for as long as is necessary.

The Mind

Tuning in to what is happening in the body during a yin practice will likely trigger a multitude of fluctuations in the mind. You may experience feelings like boredom, discomfort, or even anxiety. Try to stay with those feelings and remember everything's okay. There's no need to chastise yourself for the various thoughts and feelings that arise as you engage in this practice.

Part of maintaining stillness is accepting the impermanent nature of the thoughts that come up during the long holds. To help regulate mind chatter, return to your breath. As you slow down and deepen your breathing, you will likely discover that your mind quiets down as well.

Additionally, your relationship to your thoughts about

yourself and how they relate to your yoga practice may change the more you engage in yin. You may learn that you have the fortitude to handle a challenging pose. You may also learn that staying present and listening to the messages your body communicates during the practice leads you to become more in tune with your body off the mat as well. Yin yoga does wonders for opening the body—and it also helps us open up our mind and how we view ourselves.

Conclusion

Yoga is more than mere stretching. It exercises the body, mind, and spirit.

It's probably not news to you that yoga is perfect for your wellbeing; the modern popularity of yoga has spread that message very effectively. But now that you've learned so much about yoga and its many benefits, you have a much better idea of the reasons for that.

The truth is that yoga, and the way we practice it through meditation and the asanas, reflects how one should live life.

Think about all the times we try to rush things, desperately trying to achieve our goals in ever smaller amounts of time because the world has become so fast. That's not inherently wrong; in fact, the intentions are good—but good intentions alone don't shape us.

The only thing that can bring you closer to your goals is constant practice, introspection, and patience. Yoga is about all that.

Practicing yoga is about flexing a little bit every day for

months just to break the tightness of our body. It's about regulating our breath and mind to endure extreme bodily poses that defy our sense of balance. Lastly, it's about knowing that the best poses will require a considerable time investment.

No matter how much you rush or how hard you press, some things simply require time and repetition. Simple as that.

This is an invaluable message for most of us today. We can't afford to get carried away by the mentality of instant gratification. We're bound to crash into a stone wall of ineptitude sooner or later if we don't start doing things with care and consistency.

I hope this book has given you more than a handful of bodily poses and sequences to train your body; in truth, I hope you realize these core life precepts. They're far more valuable.

That is not to diminish the impacts of yoga on your health. If you're like me, and you work a lot of hours at the computer, you might be accustomed to the stiff feeling of your body. Some days you don't even want to sit at all. That is one perfect reason to start practicing yoga.

With just 20 minutes each day, you can breathe more life and energy into your seemingly spent body. The surge of power will allow you to achieve more, but besides this tangible surge of wellbeing, think about how good it would be to reconnect with your respiration and your thoughts every day.

We've become disconnected from our inner self. In a

single span of time we think of so many different and unrelated things that we can't even follow our own train of thought.

Yoga demands you stop for a moment, forcing you to reflect.

Indeed, yoga is truly a wonderful school of philosophy and exercise. Practicing it, and doing it honestly, with an open mind and an open heart, will get you a multitude of benefits that go far beyond stretching both of your legs parallel to the ground.

I hope this book was able to help you get acquainted with the different yoga poses.

The next step is to apply what you have learned in this book to change your life. Yoga has tremendous physical and mental health benefits. It strengthens your mind and your body. Yoga also helps keep your body fit, too. Yoga is fun, light, and challenging at the same time.

Also, it is important to consult your doctor before trying any of the poses featured in this book. If you are a beginner, it is best to start your yoga practice under the supervision of a certified yoga teacher.

Good luck yogi, your ascetic journey has just barely begun!